HEALING
MUSHROOMS

P9-CBE-550

HEALING
MUSHROOMS

· ·

A Practical and Culinary Guide to Using
Mushrooms for Whole Body Health

TERO ISOKAUPPILA

Foreword by Mark Hyman, MD

AVERY
AN IMPRINT OF PENGUIN RANDOM HOUSE
NEW YORK

AVERY

an imprint of Penguin Random House LLC
375 Hudson Street
New York, New York 10014

Copyright © 2017 Four Sigma Foods, Inc.
Illustrations copyright © Juho Heinola
Photographs copyright © Markus Karjalainen
Penguin supports copyright. Copyright fuels creativity, encourages diverse voices,
promotes free speech, and creates a vibrant culture. Thank you for buying an authorized
edition of this book and for complying with copyright laws by not reproducing, scanning,
or distributing any part of it in any form without permission. You are supporting
writers and allowing Penguin to continue to publish books for every reader.

Most Avery books are available at special quantity discounts for bulk purchase
for sales promotions, premiums, fund-raising, and educational needs.
Special books or book excerpts also can be created to fit specific needs.
For details, write SpecialMarkets@penguinrandomhouse.com.

ISBN 9780735216020

Printed in the United States of America
5   7   9   10   8   6

BOOK DESIGN BY MEIGHAN CAVANAUGH

Neither the publisher nor the author is engaged in rendering professional advice or services to the individual reader. The ideas, procedures, and suggestions contained in this book are not intended as a substitute for consulting with your physician. All matters regarding your health require medical supervision. Neither the author nor the publisher shall be liable or responsible for any loss or damage allegedly arising from any information or suggestion in this book.

The recipes contained in this book have been created for the ingredients and techniques indicated. The publisher is not responsible for your specific health or allergy needs that may require supervision. Nor is the publisher responsible for any adverse reactions you may have to the recipes contained in the book, whether you follow them as written or modify them to suit your personal dietary needs or tastes.

CONTENTS

FOREWORD

My patients are always asking me what my top superfoods are. I realize "superfood" carries a certain hype, but some foods *do* earn that status. Food is medicine. And some foods are more potent medicines than others! Food is the most powerful tool to create optimal health. Food is the most powerful drug in my arsenal, and the first I use to treat my patients.

While visiting China, I discovered folks there knew more about food's medicinal properties than I did, even after many years of research. Medicinal foods are a part of their everyday diet, and mushrooms, one of my favorite superfoods, play a huge role in Chinese medicine. These mushrooms, such as reishi, shiitake, maitake, and cordyceps, have such well-known healing powers that they are commonly referred to as functional or medicinal mushrooms. Consuming mushrooms for health benefits like energy, longevity, and immunity is a part of the everyday culture in China—unlike in the United States, where most general consumers don't know a portabello from a shiitake. This, however, is about to change.

Top mushrooms like chaga and lion's mane are trending right now in the science and medical research communities of the Western world—

and it's just the beginning. Their antiviral and anti-inflammatory properties hold great potential to combat many of our largest health problems, from cancer to diabetes and from auto-immune diseases to nervous system attacks. Current research shows that functional mushrooms have a myriad of healing properties such as inhibiting cancer cell growth, balancing excess hormones like estrogens via aromatase, and reducing chronic fatigue. And in the coming years, we're going to see even more new Western-based research published on the medicinal benefits of mushrooms.

The list of vital nutrients found in mushrooms is extensive. They are an excellent source of nutrients, such as Vitamin D, biotin, pantothenic acid, selenium, copper, and riboflavin. Vitamin D, which an estimated 50 to 75 percent of Americans are deficient in, is linked to improved cardiovascular health, hormonal regulation, and elevated mood. Biotin, or Vitamin B_7, is known to help with our skin health, nervous system, and digestive tract. Pantothenic acid, or Vitamin B_5, is often prescribed orally for inflammatory issues such as arthritis and premenstrual syndrome (PMS). Selenium can help regulate thyroid functions, and copper and riboflavin are great aids in natural energy production. With all these benefits packed into one delicate functional fungi, it's no wonder many informed people refer to mushrooms as the original superfoods.

As people gain a greater understanding of mushrooms' nutritional value, they may still lack the how-to knowledge they need to incorporate them into their daily lives. Enter Tero Isokauppila, a thirteenth-generation Finnish farmer transplanted to Venice, California, and his book, *Healing Mushrooms*. Here, Tero shares a deep knowledge about the world of mushrooms as well as creative recipes with surprising healing properties that fit today's most common dietary preferences, from vegan to paleo, ketogenic to leaky gut, and everything in between.

While mushrooms are a versatile whole food to cook with, they require special attention to flavor combinations, ingredient preparation, and know-how to ensure their unique healing properties come through in finished dishes. Tero teaches us in a simple and "funguy" way exactly how to do this. He is both entertaining and illuminating in the way he talks about the power and uses of functional mushrooms. In fact, he is truly the perfect ambassador for the mushroom kingdom.

I drink mushroom tea, cook with mushrooms such as shiitake, and make soups with wild mushrooms. While reading this book, even I was surprised by all the ways we can incorporate these healing superfoods into our daily lives without sacrificing convenience or deliciousness. Cordyceps ice cubes, lion's mane lattes, mushroom bacon, and paleo ice cream, anyone?

Read on, and you will never think about consuming mushrooms in the same way again.

—Mark Hyman, MD

A FARMING FOUNDATION

grew up in Finland on a farm that has been in my family for at least thirteen generations. Much of my youth was spent outdoors, learning from and living off the land. That may sound idyllic, and in many ways it was, but my point is not to paint a picture of my childhood as being cut from a Laura Ingalls Wilder book. Rather, I want to illuminate that it was never an option for me to not be dependent on the land on which I lived. To understand how I came to be so invested in mushrooms, how I came to be the "funguy" I so devotedly am, it's necessary to start with my childhood.

As the youngest son in a farming family, I started working basically as soon as I could walk. I cut grass, fed our calves, and could even drive a tractor by the age of five. This may sound like a lot of labor for a child, but such was the norm in farming families. While work itself was a constant guarantee, its nature depended on our daily needs. Sometimes, we spent entire days removing rocks from the land—our harvester would get jammed and often break down if we drove over a rock, so the fields needed to be cleared. This had to be done manually, so I would walk the property all day in search of obtrusive rocks to haul off to make way for harvesting. This was maybe my least favorite job, as it was really, really boring. But there were exciting jobs, too, and many days when the work did not feel like actual work at all.

For instance, there were days I spent foraging with my mother. Her farming knowledge was nurtured from practical experience that began, like mine, at an early age. She came from quite a poor background, so she didn't have a plot of family land to inherit as my father did, and started foraging as a young child partly out of necessity. As she grew up, she became increasingly interested and adept at foraging. It was the activity on our farm that she always loved best. Though her true passion lies in sourcing wild berries—I don't know that any guest has ever left our house without a parting gift in the form of a big bag of her gathered berries—she nevertheless taught me much of what I know about foraging for mushrooms.

As someone who now travels all over the world for work, I still try to forage a bit wherever I go. Foraging allows me to connect with nature and calm my mind—finding healthy, free food is really just a bonus! But none of my endeavors today quite compare to my early days as a boy in Finland, roaming our land and bringing my findings home to contribute to the meals we'd cook in our farmhouse kitchen. Now whenever I am asked how I came to initially be interested in mushrooms, the first thing that comes to mind is foraging for porcini and chanterelles in the woods on my family's farm. I can still taste the traditional dishes my mother would whip up with my finds—the creamy mushroom soup I loved or my father's favorite, steak with mushroom sauce. Of course, my interest in mushrooms when I was a child was based solely on how they tasted. I knew nothing about their health benefits, just that I loved to eat them. I had no idea of the limitless power and potential within this vast and incredible kingdom, nor did I have any inkling that mushrooms would later come to play such an enormous role in my professional and personal life.

The Turning Point

The next stepping stone on my path to the world of mycology and to uncovering the medicinal powers of mushrooms occurred when I was in college. Like many of my peers, I was interested in making some extra pocket money, so a few friends and I entered an innovation contest. Our plan to export the matsutake mushroom (also known as the pine mushroom, or *Tricholoma matsutake*), a culinary variety that often sold for more than $1,000 per pound, from Finland to Japan was the winning entry. I thought it was pretty compelling stuff (people pay that much for a nugget of fungus? Really?), but even then, I still would never have guessed how significantly mushrooms would factor in my future.

Later, as a semicompetitive runner in my twenties, I became interested in physiology as it pertained to achieving peak performance in running. Through my research and in talking to several people who worked in the health and nutrition field I was introduced to a mushroom variety called cordyceps. What I learned was an athlete's dream: cordyceps has astounding properties that make it instrumental for both increasing energy and reducing fatigue. I quickly found a reputable online source of cordyceps capsules and started pouring the capsule contents into my daily pre-run smoothies. I would start my run fifteen minutes after drinking the smoothie, and in that time frame—a mere quarter of an hour—I felt an unmistakable and remarkable surge of energy.

These days, labeling something a "superfood" is often just a means of capitalizing on a buzzy edible trend. Of course, many foods deserve such a label. But it's hard to know how exactly to consume these nutritious marvels in order to reap the alleged positive benefits. For instance, how many, say, blueberries do you need to eat and in what combination with other foods and for how long before you notice a physical difference? Another example: dark leafy greens are touted as supremely nutritious, but after eating a kale salad do you actually feel better? Like in an immediate, recognizable way? What was astounding about my first experience with cordyceps was how it affected me in clear, positive manners, almost immediately. It was like drinking a cup of coffee—how you can feel its energizing effects right after you drink it. It's a palpable sensation. That was exactly how cordyceps acted on my body. And to think that cordyceps was just one mushroom in a kingdom with more than one and a half million members! I had read research extolling mushrooms as a superfood, with the capacity to do everything from boosting immune function and improving sleep quality to lowering bad cholesterol and eliminating cancer. Now that I had experienced such incredible, beneficial effects after taking just a few capsules of cordyceps, these claims about mushrooms had a new level of merit. Imagining what else could be achieved with other varieties was mind blowing. That was my "hell yeah" mushroom moment, when I knew mushrooms were undeniably a superfood. And just like that it was official: I became a full-on funguy.

Being Called a Funguy

This is my corny way of saying that I'm wholly invested in understanding and disseminating the fungi kingdom as it relates to human health and wellness. Anyone who's on board with that crusade, and who does not take everything too seriously, gets branded a funguy as well. The name fits because even though much of the information to be gleaned from the fungi kingdom is rooted in biology and chemistry, there're plenty of ways to make it accessible, engaging, and *fun*.

Mushrooms to the Masses

My new obsession led me to research different varieties of mushrooms, and I uncovered a centuries-long history of how members of the fungi kingdom have positively affected human health and wellness. It confounded me that this wasn't information that was universally understood—how could people not know about this? How could I have not known about this? But the fact is that while East Asian cultures have a time-honored tradition of using fungi for a wide variety of benefits, their medicinal properties never really caught on in mainstream Western cultures—and in the Americas, especially. We'll get into why that might have been the case in chapter 2 of this book.

Firmly believing that everyone deserves to reap the incredible benefits that come from incorporating mushrooms into a daily wellness regimen, I founded Four Sigmatic, a superfood company, in 2012. Our dream was to popularize the consumption of medicinal mushrooms by making them accessible to everyone. Of course, mushrooms have always been available to those who were passionate enough to obtain them—many of the mushrooms we'll discuss in this book grow prolifically across the United States, and those that don't are still relatively easy to obtain with a bit of research and resourcefulness. But a problem for many would-be mushroom users is that even if someone had access to the mushrooms themselves, it didn't guarantee that they'd be able to optimally tap into the mushrooms' benefits, especially considering that many of the most potent mushrooms are not easily edible in their natural form. With Four Sigmatic, we knew we needed to make these powerful mushrooms accessible for anyone who wanted them, and to do so, we would need to make our mushroom products approachable and super user-friendly. We made it our mission to offer medicinal mushrooms to consumers in such a way that they would merely be upgrading or replacing existing habits with healthier options that contained mushrooms. Coffee proved to be a natural starting point. People love their morning cup of coffee, but some feel guilty about their caffeine habit. When coffee contains healthy chaga, reishi, or lion's mane, however, it can be transformed to a wholly nourishing ritual. Mushroom coffee became our gateway item—it's like the California roll of the fungi kingdom—and it allowed us to introduce people to mushrooms in a simple, seamless, and delicious way. We started Four Sigmatic in northern Europe, then moved the business to the United States in 2014 and launched our beverage products there in 2015. And now we're full-on living our dream of bringing mushrooms to the masses. Masses who are, incidentally, becoming increasingly hungry for alternative means to achieve optimal health and wellness.

Crusading for 'Shrooms

These days, when I tell people—strangers, friends, family members, possible love interests—that I am passionate about fungi, the reactions I get are never dull. They're confused, surprised, skeptical, intrigued. Some are even disgusted—I can practically see a cartoon bubble emerge from the head of whomever I am speaking to: "Mushrooms must be big in Finland." "Just another hipster forager." "He must be a chef!! I'll ask him about morels!" "Oh geez, is this dude going to start talking about his years following Phish?"

These are all valid reactions. People hear the word *mushroom* and often have surprisingly specific ideas of what they think the larger conversation is. And it's no shock that the reaction is often not entirely favorable. After all, mushrooms aren't intrinsically compelling to us in the way that, say, chocolate is, and people's knowledge about mushrooms is generally limited to what they cook with or eat, what they've seen growing in the woods, and what some guy named Dave sold out of his dorm room back in the day. We've all heard cautionary tales about the poisonous potential of wild mushrooms, and we've seen elation spread over the faces of world-famous chefs as they extol certain varietals of fungi in an almost evangelical manner.

The fact that mushrooms can be both poisonous and delicious is fascinating and indicative of their complexity; the kingdom is such a vast and complete entity that both the yin and the yang exist in equal measure. While we could easily write a book—or several—about culinary, poisonous, and psychedelic mushrooms, none of those varieties are what *this* book is about.

What this book is about, and what is singularly and intensely compelling about the mushrooms we focus on here, is that fungi have the capacity to change your life in an immediate, powerful, and exponentially beneficial manner. I know this because I see it happen on a daily, if not hourly, basis. Mushrooms will blow your mind, just as they did—and continue to blow—my own.

These medicinal mushrooms will balance and restore your immune system, increase oxygen flow to your cells, amp up your mental and creative acuity, regulate your blood sugar, lower your stress levels, ensure restful sleep, and cure myriad physical, emotional, and mental ailments. If you know how to use and consume even a few of the different varieties of the mushrooms discussed in this book, you will heal and recharge your body, reach your full potential, and become the very best version of you.

I know it sounds too good to be true. It sounds suspiciously like one of those nebulous "miracle" cures or like I spent a little too much time with that Dave guy back in the dorm. But trust me on this.

Trust me, because I'm someone who travels a heck of a lot for business (we're talking upward of forty trips per year). That's a lot of exposure to germs and wear and tear on the immune system—yet I haven't been sick for a single day in almost a decade.

Trust me, because I have lived in eight countries on three continents over the past ten years, and in every single place mushrooms are used in countless ways—both overt and hidden—to heal the human body and help it to flourish. Globally, we might not agree on much, but we are all on board with fungi.

Trust me, because I have studied with mycologists, chefs, and health and nutrition experts to gain so much information on mushrooms that my head could explode, but I have condensed the information and made it accessible for you with this book.

Trust me, because mushrooms are used in more than 40 percent of pharmaceuticals available on the market today (including penicillin, immunosuppressants, and several of the most prescribed anticholesterol statins on the market).

Trust me, because 92 percent of plants depend on mushroom mycelium to survive, something that is easier to fathom when you consider that 25 percent of Earth's biomass is fungi.

Trust me, because human beings and mushrooms share roughly 85 percent of the same ribosomal RNA and almost 50 percent of the same DNA—rendering many forms of fungi extremely bioavailable for the human body (i.e., able to assist in curing a wide swath of ailments and disease).

Trust me, because I was just a normal guy who stumbled into the incredible world of fungi and, knowing what I know now, can't keep this invaluable and powerful information to myself.

The fungi kingdom contains more mushrooms than have even been identified at this point, but the ten varieties we discuss in this book are tried and true powerhouses, relatively easy to find and use, and will change your life so dramatically that you'll want to go out and research others once you've experienced their effects. We'll also talk a bit about foraging, ease any fears about allergies and child safety, and assuage the skepticism of those who can't get past the unsavory origins of certain mushrooms.

Here, we've included recipes that have been developed by my business partner and chef, Lari Laurikkala, and myself. Many of these dishes are "run to your kitchen and make these now" good (including pizza, fries, and risotto), and others will require a sense of adventure (kombucha, jelly bowls, and cocktails). We had more than five hundred recipes to choose from and we are sharing the fifty we've decided are the best, not only in terms of taste but also in how they deliver the most valuable and potent properties of the mushrooms they use. Trust me once again when I say that you'll be amazed to discover how surprisingly delicious these functional mushrooms can be in desserts and beverages.

I WOULD NEVER HAVE IMAGINED that I would start a company that sells mushroom beverage powders. Drinking mushrooms? Yeah, that sounded pretty strange to me at first, too. But after years of taking supplements for various reasons—general health, athletic performance, immune support—with no identifiable results, and then experiencing firsthand the powers of these mushrooms, I knew medicinal mushrooms were my calling. Now I'm sharing what I've learned with you in this book, because above all else, I believe small changes can lead to big impact on health and wellness. And because I'm one heck of a funguy.

1

MUSHROOM LINGO

You don't need to be a chemist, mycologist, or health-and-wellness expert to understand the multitude of benefits you can experience by adding medicinal mushrooms to your life. However, the nature of the beast is that much of what we're going to talk about is rooted in chemistry and biology. Before you start having painful flashbacks involving Bunsen burners and dreaded high school science classes, rest assured that we're just giving you the basic terminology here. These definitions are not exhaustive or clinical, but rather contain the information that will be most helpful for you to reference as you use and cook your way through this book. Though we've simplified things, the science stuff can still be complicated. If something here proves elusive, just skim the definition and come back to it when the term crops up again. And want to know the best part? Even if you never understand what a polysaccharide is, the mushrooms will still work their magic.

Fungi Kingdom

Depending on whom you ask and where you live, there are currently five or six recognized kingdoms of living organisms on Earth. (In the United States, the six typically accepted kingdoms are *Animalia, Plantae, Fungi, Protista, Archaebacteria*, and *Eubacteria*.) Of course, the more we learn, the more kingdoms may emerge. This probability for further discovery rings especially true considering that for a long time, fungi were classified as part of the plant kingdom. But as fungi were studied, it became apparent that they deserved to be classified in their own kingdom, as they actually share more similarities with animals than with plants (in fact, fungi and animals are part of the same superkingdom: *Opisthokonta*). Like humans and other animals, fungi are *heterotrophic,* meaning they are dependent on other organisms for obtaining nutrients. Of course, our eating patterns differ, as fungi absorb their nutrients by releasing enzymes to break down food sources, which they will then sprout from. There are estimated to be more than 1.5 million types of fungi, and more than 90 percent of those varieties have not yet been recognized or named. The ten medicinal and culinary mushrooms we are focusing on are but an infinitesimal portion of the vast fungi kingdom.

So what do you really need to know? Let's start with these three things about the fungi kingdom: First, not all fungi are mushrooms, but all mushrooms are fungi. Under the fungi umbrella are also molds like those found on cheeses like Camembert and Gorgonzola and those used for their antibiotic properties, such as penicillin. There are yeasts like those used to make bread and beer. Second, remember that fungi require external food sources. Unlike plants, which make their own food through photosynthesis, many fungi are *saprotrophs*, which means they obtain nutrients by consuming dead and decaying organisms. Third, compared to the plant and animal kingdoms, the fungi kingdom as a whole has been far less studied, which makes it an exciting platform for exploration and also lends credence as to why the astonishing superpowers of medicinal mushrooms have been largely unknown to the masses in Western cultures. And while roughly 40 percent of all pharmaceuticals contain fungi in some form, we're still only scratching the surface of the power that fungi can provide. So what's the takeaway? By reading this book, you're on the cutting edge of significant scientific and health revelations. How about that?

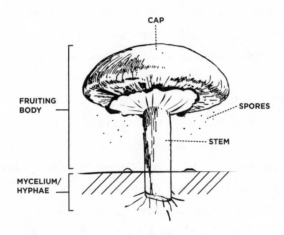

The anatomy of a shiitake mushroom

Mycelium

Think of mycelium as the root system of mushrooms. Mycelium forms when mushroom *fruiting bodies* release spores that then germinate into *hyphae:* tubular, feathery filaments that grow in the form of an underground web, often of enormous proportions, just like the roots of a tree. Any time you walk over an area where you see mushroom fruiting bodies—and even in areas with no signs of mushrooms at all—you are walking over fungi mycelium. In fact, if you happen to be walking over areas of eastern Oregon, you might be walking over a mycelium that is considered to be the largest living organism on Earth. This honey mushroom (*Armillaria solidipes*) mycelium spans about 2,400 acres (roughly

1,665 football fields), weighs between 7,500 and 35,000 tons, and is between 2,000 and 8,000 years old. It's pretty mind blowing when you think about it.

The mycelium is the most environmentally important part of the mushroom. It acts as a fishing net, surrounding and penetrating the root systems of plants and trees, absorbing water and other nutrients from the surrounding environment and transferring them to the plants, allowing them to thrive. As such, it can be said that the medicinal properties of many plants are contingent on the mushrooms that grow near them. The mycelium also releases the enzymes that break down dead or decaying plant life. The mycelium absorbs the nutrients to form a *fruiting body*, and the plant is decomposed into healthy soil ready to welcome the growth of new flora.

It may sound a little woo-woo at first, but mycelium can actually help plants communicate among themselves. The mycelial network is a sort of underground web of information made of woodlike matter called *chiton*, and this network is often referred to as the "original Internet." It shares information about possible intruders and pathogens, and can create a fungal defense system by releasing toxins to fight them off. Mycelium shares information as to where nutrients like water, phosphorus, and nitrogen are to help nearby plants flourish, and in return, the fungi will absorb energy in the form of carbs from the plants. This mutually beneficial relationship with fungi and plants is so powerful that even plants that are entirely different species can exchange nutrients with one another via this mycelial network.

Fruiting Body

This is the part of the fungi that grows aboveground, the part we typically call the "mushroom," though it is in fact only a part of the whole (see diagram on page 13). The fruiting body is often edible and is frequently found in the classic shape of a stem with a cap (though its appearance depends on the type of mushroom you are dealing with—some varieties have fruiting bodies that look quite different from what we think of as a classic mushroom shape, and you'll learn more about that in chapter 3). While the mycelium is the part of the fungi that is most important to the well-being of the plant kingdom, the fruiting body is the part that is most beneficial for humans. With a few exceptions, most mushrooms are annuals, meaning once a year, the mycelium continually produces fruiting bodies. An important idea to keep in mind is that though we call all the mushroom varieties we're introducing you to "mushrooms," what we're really referring to are their fruiting bodies. While each part of the mushroom plays a valuable role in nature, the fruiting body is the part used in cooking and predominantly for health and wellness.

SUSTAINABLE FORAGING

If you're foraging for mushrooms, feel free to gather with abandon, but do try to leave a few mushrooms where you found them. Even though research suggests that whether you pick all the mushrooms or none of them has little effect on the growth or health of the mycelium, leaving some mushrooms will ensure that spores are released for future growth. Note that this new growth will not necessarily happen in the exact same spot every year—spores are inevitably spread by wind, water, animals, birds, insects, and even the bottoms of your shoes. The good thing is that slightly older, past-their-prime mushrooms will still release spores, so leaving those for regeneration is an easy foraging best practice.

Spores

Also called fungal seeds, these are the asexual reproductive units of the fungi's fruiting body that are released from its gills or pores (the pores are also referred to as *stoma*). While fruiting bodies often produce thousands—and up to trillions, depending on their size—of spores *a day*, only a small fraction of those spores will germinate and eventually develop into a fruiting body. Mushroom spores are everywhere—they're floating in the air around you and living on your pillowcases; with every breath you take, you breathe in up to ten spores. But don't worry, they're completely harmless.

Here's a fun example that illustrates just how many spores mushrooms release: According to the calculations of acclaimed mycologist David Arora, the amount of spores produced by a single giant puffball mushroom (*Calvatia gigantea*) could circle the earth at its equator. And even more incredibly, if each of these spores were to grow into a giant puffball, they could be arranged in a line that would extend to the sun and back (that's almost 186 million miles), and they'd have a collective weight eight hundred times greater than planet Earth. These calculations may not be entirely accurate, but what is 100% certain is that the number of spores puffball mushrooms produce is mind-boggling.

There are two other cool things to know about mushroom spores: First, they're made of chitin, which is among the hardest naturally occurring substances on Earth. Second, spores are the fastest live organisms on the planet. Granted, the speed at which they travel only ever applies to very short distances, but they're still incredibly fast. For example, the *Pilobolus* mushroom releases its spores into the air at a rate of 20,000 G's of force. Other studies indicate that some fruiting bodies could even explode their spores at a rate of more than 180,000 G's! By comparison, fighter pilots can withstand roughly 5 to 9 G's, and these are people who are trained to be the best in the world at bearing large amounts of force.

Saprotrophs

This term describes organisms that feed on the dead or decaying matter of other organisms. Most fungi are saprotrophs (those that aren't are *symbionts*, meaning they obtain their nutrients from living rather than dead organisms). Many of the medicinal mushrooms we'll introduce you to, such as reishi, enoki, shiitake, maitake, and oyster mushrooms, grow mainly on dead trees. The *fruiting bodies* of these fungi sprout from the trees once their *mycelium* have absorbed the tree's nutrients.

This eating pattern is remarkable because fungi essentially recycle plant life by absorbing the dead matter and redistributing the plant's nutrients. Rather than simply being left to rot, the decaying tree will ultimately be broken down by fungi to become nutrient-rich soil. It's an impressive symbiotic relationship.

THE FINAL SUIT

Plants are not the only things that get broken down by fungi. Due to their ability to recycle a wide range of organic materials, mushrooms are now starting to be used in human burial suits. These suits are designed to filter out the toxins we've collected during our life span and help decompose our bodies, transforming us into healthy soil that will foster future life.

Extremophile

As the name implies, these are organisms that can prosper in extreme environments. Fungi are extremophiles, having earned this classification due to their ability to survive and thrive in a wide range of inhospitable environments and severe atmospheric conditions. They can withstand the low-air-pressure environment of outer space (several forms of fungi lived in the Russian-operated Mir Space Station during its twenty-year existence), the scorching desert heat, the below-freezing temperatures of Antarctica, and even the radioactivity of nuclear reactors. In fact, it's said that mushrooms were in contact with radiation during the Chernobyl Nuclear Disaster of 1986, yet they emerged entirely unscathed. Fungi can also live underwater (currently a vastly unexplored arena in the fungi kingdom; my guess is that many future fungi discoveries will arise from aquatic-based research). Being the extremophiles that they are, fungi have existed on Earth for an estimated 1,300 million-plus years, initially obtaining nutrients from rocks until plants began to grow on the planet.

CLEANSING THE AIR, ONE 'SHROOM AT A TIME

Saprotrophs have the ability to decompose synthetic pollutants such as the pesticide DDT, plastics, and possibly the worst manufactured compounds of all time: Venomous Agent X (VX) and sarin gas, which are used as chemical warfare weapons. Since these nasty man-made toxins are created by combining molecules that don't exist in nature, they're often believed to be indestructible by natural (or any) means. It makes you wonder: If mushrooms can counteract the effects of something as extreme and dangerous as a compound used for chemical warfare, they have incredible potential for protecting us from the many less-powerful yet ubiquitous toxins we encounter every day—such as automobile exhaust.

Adaptogens

These are naturally occurring nontoxic substances that protect the body from stress by stabilizing and optimizing its physiological functions. Adaptogens boost immunity, protect you from disease, and promote overall health and wellness. Many plants and mushrooms—such as ginseng root, holy basil, cordyceps, and reishi—are well known for their adaptogenic properties. To qualify as an adaptogen, a mushroom must help the body in a nonspecific way. That last bit is important because rather than serving a single targeted purpose, adaptogenic mushrooms will adapt their healing properties to whatever your body specifically needs at a given time in order to restore you to peak functionality. Think of adaptogens this way: You know that good friend who comes over to your house to vent after she's had a bad day, but sees that you're over the moon about some terrific news and promptly adjusts her demeanor to celebrate your happiness with you? That's what an adaptogen does in the human body— it senses what the body needs and alters its behavior in whatever way necessary to foster peak health.

Immunomodulators

These work similarly to adaptogens, but immunomodulators only relate to your immune system. When your defenses are down, you become susceptible to catching a cold or succumbing to a more serious illness or disease. By contrast, when your body tries to address issues that are not even there and begins to attack itself, you experience inflammation or even develop an autoimmune disorder. Your body will turn against you when it is confused—either by signaling a hypoactive or hyperactive defense response—so immunomodulators play a critical role in keeping your immune system stable and consistent. All the medicinal mushrooms you will meet in chapter 3 have immunomodulating capacities.

So how exactly does the immunomodulating process work? Here's a simple analogy: Say you're driving on a long stretch of highway, and you set your cruise control to 60 mph. Whenever you go uphill and need a bit of a boost, the car will automatically adjust to maintain the speed set by the cruise control. When you go downhill, the car will adjust in the opposite direction to ensure you are still operating at that smooth and steady 60 mph. What cruise control is to driving, immunomodulators are to the immune system—regulating everything to ensure a smooth, stable ride.

Polysaccharides

It's time to get a little bit science-y. Polysaccharides are water-soluble chemical compounds made up of chains of complex (*poly*) carbohydrates (*saccharides*). Three common polysaccharides are starch, glycogen, and cellulose. All are composed of glucose, or sugar. Starch and glycogen function as short-term energy stores in plants and animals, while cellulose is the main component of plant cell walls and is also the most plentiful organic molecule on Earth. While they're the most recognized and prevalent of all polysaccharides, they don't necessarily offer any special properties for human health, and that may be why you had not previously considered polysaccharides to be incredibly beneficial to overall health and wellness. But they are, especially when you consider the unique and extremely complex polysaccharides found in fungi. These compounds act as immunomodulators—with each different strain having specific positive effects on your health. For example, the maitake mushroom contains a polysaccharide that has been shown to lower blood pressure, stabilize blood sugar, and lower cholesterol, while the shiitake mushroom has a polysaccharide that has proven to be more aggressive at targeting HIV-infected cells than the most-used HIV-treatment pharmaceutical on the market and also effectively stimulates antibodies that counteract the effects of hepatitis B. All the polysaccharides found in the medicinal mushrooms we discuss in this book activate the generation of cells that kill foreign pathogens. While there are many different types of polysaccharides, it is the *beta-glucans* we focus on for their positive immunomodulating benefits.

FOR THE CARB CONSCIOUS

Reading about the positive benefits of the polysaccharides in mushrooms may cause a warning bell to go off in many heads due to the carb-phobic eating trends of the past decade or so. However, remember that not all carbohydrates are created equal. While simple carbs such as those in white sugar, pasta, and refined flour break down quickly—causing that "spike and crash" of energy—more complex polysaccharide chains like those found in whole grains, legumes, and mushrooms provide the lasting energy your body requires to function at optimal levels. In fact, our cells actually need to be fueled by these good chains of "many sugars" to effectively communicate with one another. Research has shown that amino acids help our cells communicate with one another via chemical signals, but new research has demonstrated that this communication requires polysaccharides, too. There's nothing to worry about, anyway, because despite the essential polysaccharides they contain and all the attention we rightfully give to these carby-compounds, mushrooms are lower in carbohydrates (and calories) than pretty much any other vegetable. Rest assured that mushrooms are an entirely suitable choice even for those on low-carb, low-glycemic, or ketogenic diets.

Beta-Glucans

These are a type of polysaccharide, so-classified due to the particular way the sugar molecules are connected in the polysaccharide chain. Just as all mushrooms are fungi but not all fungi are mushrooms, all beta-glucans are polysaccharides, but not all polysaccharides are beta-glucans. Beta-glucans are perhaps most instrumental in their potential to reduce cancerous cells that have invaded the body. Among other things, the proliferation of cancerous cells often results in an overactive immune response, so the immunomodulating properties of beta-glucans will re-regulate the immune system, enabling it to better stave off the disease. They do this in part by binding to macrophage, natural killer (NK), and other white blood cells in the body to trigger an appropriate immune response from cells that specifically target cancerous growths. Beta-glucans also stimulate the creation of immune stem cells in bone marrow and stimulate other white blood cells (such as NK cells) to release anti-cancer molecules throughout the body, so the immune system is equipped to ward off and reduce cancerous invasions as well as mitigate the effects of chemotherapy and radiation. For these reasons, scientists have classified beta-glucans as "biological response modifiers" and have praised them because they are perhaps the only identified substance that boosts immunity without ever pushing the immune system to overreact.

Still, research on beta-glucans and how they affect cancer, while substantial, is very much in its nascent stages. Doubtless you'll be hearing a lot more about how these compounds work to reduce and eliminate cancer as both an alternative and a complement to Western treatments.

The body does not produce beta-glucans on its own, so they must be consumed in the foods we eat. Though they exist in many foods (oats and barley, for example), the best way for your body to obtain beta-glucans is through mushrooms (in extract form) because of their high concentration and the abundance of research on their bioavailability. The beta-glucan formation varies from mushroom to mushroom. For example, the mushrooms we cover in this book each contain their own unique strains of beta-glucans, and each strain has specific healing properties—some can dramatically reduce the symptoms of asthma, while others do wonders to mitigate the effects of heart disease—but regardless, all work to restore and promote peak immune function. You'll learn more about beta-glucans in the next chapter.

Terpenoids

Also known as terpenes, terpenoids are common examples of fat-soluble chemical compounds with proven antiviral and antibacterial properties. There are other similar fat-soluble compounds, but these are the most well-known. Terpenoids work as anti-infectious agents by stimulating the destruction of bacteria and viruses that invade the body and by preventing the immune system from overreacting. Terpenoids also play a powerful role in balancing your hormone levels. But perhaps most important are their anti-inflammatory properties.

Inflammation is the body's natural healing response, but too much inflammation can be detrimental. For example, when you catch a cold, the redness in your nose and throat is your body's inflammatory response to the virus. The redness indicates increased blood flow and more permeable blood vessels, which allow healing white blood cells to enter the inflamed areas to attack the virus. Sometimes, these healing cells are sent in higher numbers than needed, so the surrounding areas also come under attack, creating new, possibly harmful areas of inflammation around the original area being targeted. If too many cells are allowed to fight the invader, the response becomes counterproductive, and this additional inflammation in the nasal and throat passages lowers your ability to breathe. A major issue with over-the-counter (OTC) drugs is that while they are effective at reducing unwanted additional inflammation, they also prevent white blood cells from doing their job on the original inflamed areas. The beauty of terpenoids, however, is that they allow white blood cells to attack foreign invaders, but they don't allow them to proliferate unnecessarily.

THE SECRET BEHIND EUCALYPTUS

While the anti-inflammatory properties of terpenoids have also proven effective in reducing cholesterol buildup in the arteries, inhibiting histamine response to seasonal allergies, and reducing chronic inflammation on a cellular level, there's a reason we're using the common cold as an example here. Terpenoids are actually a form of "original medicine"—just think about the long history of inhaling and using eucalyptus for its ability to fend off and alleviate cold symptoms. It turns out that eucalyptus leaves contain terpenoids—how about that?

Dual Extraction

Also known as double extraction, this is the method used to obtain the maximum health benefits from mushrooms. It's used especially with varieties like chaga, reishi, turkey tail, and others that can't simply be sautéed in a pan or easily ground into a powder. It's a two-step process: first, an alcohol extraction pulls out the fat-soluble compounds (creating a tincture), and second, a hot-water extraction pulls out the water-soluble compounds from the fungi (creating a decoction).

In the alcohol extraction, the mushrooms are soaked in alcohol, often for multiple weeks, to release the fat-soluble compounds, like the terpenoids. Fat-soluble compounds are impervious to hot water, so alcohol is necessary to draw them out. The mushrooms are then dropped into hot water to release the water-soluble polysaccharides. The water needs to be hot because polysaccharides are essentially sugars—this makes sense when you consider how much more readily sugar dissolves in hot water than in cold. These two extractions can then be combined or consumed individually. You can also easily evaporate the alcohol from the tincture if you don't wish to consume it, or you can use vinegar or glycerol as the solvent instead. Regardless of which solvent you use, the dual-extraction method is key to obtaining the maximum health benefits from fungi.

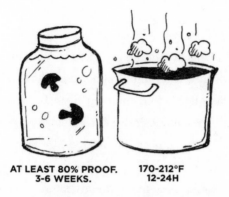

AT LEAST 80% PROOF.   170-212°F
3-6 WEEKS.   12-24H

Dual extraction is a lengthy process.

Fermentation

This is a chemical process involving bacteria, yeast, or other fungal microorganisms to break down substances. For instance, *saccharomyces*, a type of yeast, is the key ingredient needed to produce wine and beer, both of which are fermented beverages. Sauerkraut is an example of a fermented food. The process used to make sauerkraut is called lactofermentation, where "lacto" refers to the lactic acid bacteria (also known as probiotics). These bacteria work in conjunction with yeast or other fungi to convert raw food into a more easily digestible form while also releasing and stabilizing the food's nutrients and prohibiting the growth of harmful bacteria.

In the case of sauerkraut, cabbage is combined with water and salt (also known as a brine) in a sterile glass jar, then sealed and left in a warm environment for a few days. During this time, the brine allows the bacteria that naturally exist on the cabbage to convert the sugars in the cabbage to lactic acid, which then acts as a natural preservative. Other lactofermented foods include kombucha, sourdough bread, kimchi, miso, and some yogurts.

Mycotoxin

Here *myco* refers to mushrooms (or anything relating to fungi) and *toxins* refer to substances that are organic but poisonous to humans. Mycotoxins tend to be unhealthy molds that enter our lives through food and our living environment. These undesirable fungi include black mold (*Stachybotrys*), the stuff home-renovation horror stories are made of, and *aflatoxins,* which are chemicals produceed by the *Aspergillus* genus of molds and can be found on many commonly eaten foods like grains, nuts, seeds, legumes, beans, coffee, and cacao. A common theory among those studying mycology is that mycotoxins are fungi that exist to regulate or mitigate the effects of other, "rival" fungi. This notion is easier to understand when you consider a fungus like *candida*, a yeast infection caused by bad mold that can best be eliminated by good bacteria like the lactic acid found in kimchi and sauerkraut. The major takeaway here is to remember that not all fungi are good, and the bad can be pervasive and common. It's important not to confuse the two.

THERE'S ONE LAST DEFINITION to consider, though we decided not to formally write it up as we recognize our inability to be objective on the matter. But here's the thing: *mycophobia* is out there. This distrust, fear, and even abhorrence of mushrooms is a reality, and we talk about it quite a bit with our mushroom-minded contemporaries. Admittedly, we also sometimes joke about it—to us, it seems absurd. Most who are afflicted with mycophobia have a societally induced, learned aversion to mushrooms. And this is a relatively common condition, as various members of the fungi kingdom have long been misunderstood, branded as rotten, poisonous, and unclean. The real shame is that these presumptions have done us all a disservice, as they've resulted in the powerful medicinal properties and healing potential of mushrooms to be largely overlooked in Western culture. As with anything else, it's about arming yourself with the right information. Fortunately, the recent rise of mushroom popularity in both the culinary and health-and-wellness spheres is helping our cause. To all you mycophobics out there, we're here to help, one medicinal mushroom at a time.

2

MUSHROOMS IN THE MAINSTREAM

Whether you're interested in alternative healing, closely follow health trends, or have a friend who's recently been raving about the wonders of chaga tea, you're probably well aware that mushrooms are having a real moment. It's pretty incredible that the exploration of the vast potential of mushrooms is now extending beyond the limits of the health-and-wellness sphere and permeating mainstream society. The question *"Why now?"* is one I field with some regularity. It's a good question. Especially when you consider that mushrooms have been on the planet for approximately 1.3 billion years—they're possibly the first organisms that existed on dry land—meaning they've essentially always been a part of life. So why haven't we taken advantage of their powerful health properties until now?

In short, some cultures *have* consistently used fungi for health, healing, general well-being, and so much more. Asian and Slavic cultures have relied on mushrooms for myriad beneficial purposes for centuries. However, depending on the country or region in question, using mushrooms went out of style in the mainstream and became limited to those who were passionate or curious enough to learn about the different varieties and seek them out. Obviously, the fungi kingdom wasn't entirely shunned since some varieties of mushrooms, like button mushrooms and morels, have maintained relatively consistent popularity in the culinary sphere, and certain fungi are essential to making wine, beer, bread, and other dietary "staples," but in general, people did stop using mushrooms in a medicinal, healing sense. We seemed to collectively forget that mushrooms are a superfood, and for centuries the Western world neglected to tap into the powers that could potentially alleviate, eliminate, or reverse illness, mental decline, environmental damage, and so much more.

Many theories attempt to explain why mushrooms dropped off the radar. Some of these explanations seem at least partially plausible, but like with most things, it was probably a combination of events that led to the lasting mycophobia embedded in Western cultures.

One theory is that historically, women served the role of community doctors and used mushrooms (along with other natural foodstuffs) as holistic remedies and healing agents. It's possible that some of these healers tapped into the hallucinogenic properties of psychedelic mushrooms, making them appear to possess supernatural powers. These women were branded as witches and shunned from society—or worse, hanged or killed—across Europe and the United States. Perhaps it was these witch hunts that led to women across Western cultures to eradicate all knowledge of mushrooms and their medicinal properties.

Another theory explaining why mushrooms fell out of favor concerns the common, understandable fear of toxic molds. We've all heard shocking news reports of "black mold" or heard home renovation horror stories involving the uncovering of a noxious mold that led to both an exponential uptick in construction costs and a host of health concerns. With molds and mushrooms both falling under the fungi umbrella, it's possible that people opted to completely avoid anything in the fungi family, not realizing that some molds are completely harmless, just as very few mushrooms are actually poisonous.

But it's the urban myth type of story that has likely played the biggest part in pushing mushrooms out of the realm of the acceptable. Though a tiny percentage of mushrooms that grow in the wild are fatal if consumed (we're talking five, maybe six types out of the more than ten thousand known varieties), it's possible that at some point, someone somewhere plucked a poisonous fruiting body from the woods, popped it into his or her mouth, and fell ill or died. It's a terrible situation to consider, and since it is unlikely that whoever witnessed to such an episode would have known which mushroom was the culprit, it was easier to malign all mushrooms. They say it only takes one bad apple to spoil the bunch, so one toxic tale could have been ruinous for our collective perception of mushrooms. These are the types of stories that only gain momentum over time, further diminishing the possibility of mushroom acceptance.

There's also the obvious fact that mushrooms look a little eccentric and grow out of all sorts of strange, even unsavory places, so it's not all that surprising that people have long possessed an inherent fear of them. They sprout out of cow dung, they mar your beautiful green lawn after a heavy rain, and they flourish in the dankest, darkest of corners. Mushrooms are often sold covered in dirt, and they become very slimy very quickly and can be unappetizingly spongy in texture. Though not all varieties of mushrooms, bacteria, yeast, or mold are safe to consume, it's unfortunately the bad, sad stories that stick in the case of fungi.

Mushrooms are also just plain mysterious. They're treated like vegetables, but unlike other vegetables, certain varieties can make you hallucinate, and in extreme cases, possibly kill you. No one is tripping after eating a helping of broccoli, and when a neighbor stops by with a basket of summer squash, no one wonders if the squash will lead to their demise.

When something is not easily placed into a recognizable category with defined limits, it can be frightening. Many people choose to avoid that which they do not understand. People might think, "Sure, that mushroom could cure my breast cancer, but could it also cause hallucinations? What if I get a 'bad' batch?" Mushroom misinformation has been strung together with rather random facts to make a confusing patchwork of often contradictory information.

So, for a host of reasons—some folkloric, some historical, some socially derived, and some just inferred—mushrooms have remained a significant part of Eastern cultures while falling off in the West. While we may not be able to pinpoint precisely why it came about, once mycophobia arrived, it stuck around.

But times, they are a-changin'. The main reason for this new outlook is that the collective state of our health is about as bad as it's ever been. People are sicker than ever. With the upsurge in incidences of cancer, autoimmune diseases, obesity, and type 2 diabetes, as well as allergies and various skin issues, people are increasingly seeking alternative means to regain their health. And they're beginning to realize that taking more and more prescribed medications comes at a cost that's not just financial in nature. To that end, some heartening news is that the medicinal mushroom market has seen an increase from about $6 billion in 1999 to upward of $18 billion in 2014—clearly, people are starting to get it.

It's also worth considering that like most trends, food trends are cyclical. In the United States, some of the biggest food "trends" include eating local, seasonal foods. Mushrooms are "on trend" in so many ways—they are naturally low in sugar, gluten-free, high in nutrients, and are an excellent vegetarian/vegan meat substitute. They're incredibly versatile when it comes to cooking, and because of this, are heavily featured in Paleo, primal, and plant-based diets. Other trends, like the excitement around kombucha over the past several years, gave way to a surging interest in fermented foods in general (like sauerkraut and kimchi), all of which depend on fungi to flourish. And because they grow in abundance just about everywhere on the planet, incorporating mushrooms into your cooking is possible no matter where you live.

When my own research into medicinal mushrooms was going full tilt, back when I started Four Sigmatic in 2012, only the few odd mycophiles and hard-core mushroom fans were interested in what we were doing. Even in 2014, when we brought the business to the United States, we were operating in a very small, specialized market. It was growing steadily, but at a super-slow pace. As we presented our new company, we heard just about every mushroom joke in the book. While some were funny, they merely illustrated that the vast majority of people had no idea what mushrooms could really do for them. Trying to sell mushroom powders as a healthy superfood meant working a niche category within a niche market. It was a tough sell.

What a difference a few years can make, though. Since launching in the United States, our products' popularity has grown across so many types of people, from mycophiles and health nuts to professional athletes and Hollywood actors. Giant food companies are becoming more and more interested in tapping into the powers of medicinal mushrooms. This shift is remarkable, and it's just the beginning. So to answer that initial question—why now? Because fungi are our future, and people are finally ready to get on board.

3

MEET THE MUSHROOMS

There are an estimated 1.5 million species in the fungi kingdom (many of them still unclassified). That's about six times more than the number of plants in the world—and more than ten thousand of them are mushrooms. Just trying to wrap your head around this information is an overwhelming task. The good news is that if you start exploring medicinal mushrooms by getting to know our top ten varieties, you'll reap a multitude of life-changing benefits.

In fact, these ten mushrooms are some of the most astoundingly untapped superfoods in the world. Everyone from children to the elderly can enjoy them safely (all the mushrooms discussed here are nonhallucinogenic and completely nontoxic) and can deliver amazing benefits. While no book in the world could fully detail the myriad powers of each mushroom, the information on the following ten will be a valuable reference and cheat sheet for you to use as you travel on your medicinal mushroom journey. Later, we'll delve into how you can cook with each of the mushrooms using our approachable recipes. From mushroom tea to mushroom cheesecake, your kitchen game will soon be putting the "fun" in "fungi."

So why these ten? Because these are the powerhouse players when it comes to accessible mushrooms in the fungi kingdom. When and if you decide to venture further into the world of mushrooms, knowing about the ten presented here will be a solid foundation from which to work. Even if you choose to focus on just one or two, you'll still be doing your body wonders in terms of optimizing immune function, achieving hormonal balance, reducing stress, and introducing antiviral, antibacterial, and anti-inflammatory agents to your immune system. Using these mushrooms will quickly translate into you feeling and looking better.

Now that you're hooked, let's meet the mushrooms.

FORAGING

To get your hands on these mushrooms, you don't need to become a master forager. We provide a number of reputable sources for purchasing all of them in our shopping guide (page 189), but if you're really interested in foraging, turn to your local mycological association for guidance. Almost every major city has one these days. You could also head to your favorite farmers' market and talk to the mushroom vendors; they can usually connect you with a local forager who can take you under his or her wing. We've chosen not to dive too deeply into foraging because mushroom availability varies from location to location, and toxic mushrooms have enough lookalikes that hands-on experience is significantly more beneficial. Once you get out there, you shouldn't have too much trouble identifying the mushrooms we include here. It's worth noting that most of the varieties we discuss grow on trees, and very, very few tree mushrooms are poisonous.

A Note on Side Effects and Dosages

We recommend that the use of medicinal mushrooms be strictly monitored for those on antibiotics, anticoagulants, certain diabetes drugs, and intravenous glucose. Since medicinal mushrooms are potent whole foods and support the body in blood circulation and blood sugar control problems, using them alongside particular drugs intended for the same purposes may cause unexpected results, or an unwanted "doubling up" on treatment. For these conditions, mushrooms may still be very beneficial; however, it is important to discuss all usage of medicinal mushrooms with your doctor and to start slowly and incrementally increase your dosage. Also, while these mushrooms are generally regarded as safe by health care professionals, if you are pregnant or regularly taking prescription medication(s), it is essential that you consult your doctor before consuming them. Though overdosing should not be an issue with either commercially available products or mushrooms used in a culinary capacity, it is still important to note that none of the information presented here is intended to be a substitute for professional medical advice, diagnosis, or treatment of any kind.

	GOOD	BETTER	BEST

	EFFECTIVE DOSAGE CHART		
DUAL-EXTRACTION	0.5g / 0.02oz	1g / 0.04oz	1.5g / 0.06oz
HOT WATER EXTRACTION (WATER TO MUSHROOM RATIO 9:1)	1g / 0.04oz	2g / 0.07oz	3g / 0.12oz
DRY MUSHROOMS	10g / 0.35oz	20g / 0.7oz	30g / 1oz
FRESH MUSHROOMS	90g / 3.2oz	180g / 6.4oz	270g / 9.6oz

These are rough estimates that vary per mushroom source and type. For example, **reishi** has less water than **shiitake** and wildcrafted **chaga** is more powerful than cultivated.

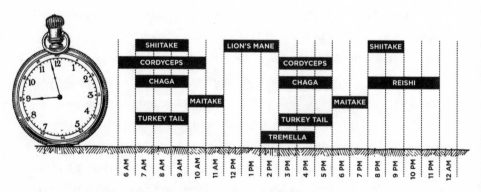

A suggested timeline showing when to take each mushroom during the day.

Mushroom Trivia Tidbit

Pharmacists in countries like Switzerland and France are required to learn mushroom identification as part of their job. Pretty telling, huh?

Reishi [rā-shē] / *Ganoderma lucidum*

USE REISHI TO

- Sleep better
- Stress less
- Cure seasonal allergies

I start many a mushroom conversation by talking about reishi, or *lingzhi*, as it is known in Chinese medicine. Among mycologists and other mushroom enthusiasts—myself included—reishi is considered the "queen of mushrooms." It's earned this moniker because of how it revitalizes the entire body (something all mushrooms do to an extent, but reishi's particularly magical in this sense) and has been revered as a miracle elixir since the days when it was reserved for use only by emperors and other royalty in ancient China. In fact, reishi was so esteemed that in ancient scroll paintings, it was depicted as the "bridge between Earth and Heaven." Other nicknames for this regal fungus include "mushroom of immortality," "mushroom of spiritual potency," and "ruler of herbs."

Reishi has been used in traditional Chinese medicine for at least two thousand years, with the first known written records dating from the Han Dynasty (206 BC to AD 220). In the original textbook of traditional Chinese medicine, written by the great Shennong ("The Divine Farmer," who is commonly recognized as the founder of Chinese medicine), reishi was ranked highest among 365 healing plants and fungi. Historically used as a source of longevity and vitality, reishi is one of the most well-studied and widely researched of the mushrooms we present here.

Reishi has the ability to boost the body's immune system to protect it against pathogens like viruses, bacteria, and parasites. Even when pathogens aren't present, an optimally functioning immune system will exponentially increase your overall health and wellness, to the point where you can witness the effects of aging being reversed—both physically and cognitively.

So how does reishi do *all* this and so much more? Let's look at longevity first. The compounds in reishi work both externally and internally to keep you looking young by reducing dermal oxidation (which is when proteins on the skin are damaged, causing wrinkles and other signs of aging) and protecting your cellular DNA and mitochondria from oxidant damage as well, allowing you to remain energized, alert, and feeling refreshed. Reishi's triterpenes (a type of terpenoid) also improve circulation, which helps with every bodily function from your mental capacities to physical appearance.

In addition to its various macro- and micronutrients, reishi is made up of polysaccharides and triterpenes. The polysaccharides (particularly the beta-glucans) act as immunomodulators. Reishi's adaptogenic properties help to stabilize your immune system so that it operates at its full potential. Reishi's polysaccharides have also been credited with lowering blood pressure, stabilizing blood sugar, lowering cholesterol, and inhibiting tumor growth in some cancers.

Another major benefit of reishi, and what truly puts it in a class of its own, is how it works to achieve hormonal balance. The specific triterpene compounds in reishi fruiting bodies support and balance the endocrine system. When you have an optimally functioning hormonal system (and surprisingly few do—for a slew of reasons including the impact of environmental toxins and the overprescribing of prescription medications, among a host of other factors), your body can relax and recover during the night as it is meant to. Taking reishi will not only increase your quality and duration of deep, restful sleep but will also allow you to function at peak levels during waking hours.

Two of reishi's most prevalent triterpenes are sterols and ganoderic acids. Sterols have been shown to lower cholesterol by impeding the absorption of cholesterol in the body, helping to improve blood circulation and heart health, and have also proven in medical studies to increase life-spans by more than 10 percent. Ganoderic acids have been shown to improve oxygen flow, boost liver functionality, and effectively inhibit histamine response, thus greatly helping those who experience seasonal allergies (see box).

REISHI IN ACTION

One of the most powerful ways I've seen reishi in action was with one of my colleagues who suffered from severe seasonal allergies for weeks every spring. When exposed to allergens, the human body releases histamines, which then cling to cells and cause them to swell and leak fluid—hence the sneezing and runny noses that accompany an increase of pollen in the air. He started taking just 1,000 milligrams of reishi daily (in the form of a dual-extracted powder dissolved into liquid), and almost immediately, his allergy symptoms disappeared entirely. It was extraordinary that in just a couple of days of consuming the equivalent of two teaspoons of this mushroom medicine, he was functioning like a normal person again, completely immune to pollen's crippling effects. That was nearly four years ago, and thanks to reishi, he can now literally wake up and smell the roses every spring.

Reishi is identified by its shiny, plastic-looking fruiting body. It almost looks fake, like a mushroom that belongs on a stage set, which is how it earned another of its nicknames, "the varnished conk" (conk is another name for the fruiting body of some tree-consuming fungi). It grows primarily on dead or dying eastern hemlock trees and ranges in color from black to purple to red. Red reishi is most commonly used in medicinal capacities because of the higher number of polysaccharides it appears to contain (though the most extensive research to date has been on the red and black varieties, so new information could be uncovered as reishi continues to be studied). Reishi is often confused with one of its (less powerful) cousins, *Ganoderma applanatum*, also known as artist's conk. Artist's conk is a more common variety, and while it has many of the same properties as reishi, the medicinal benefits are not nearly as potent (but it may affect your subconscious in a way that reishi does not—after consuming it, many people have reported having some crazy dreams!). Artist's conk is distinguished from reishi by its more subdued brown-and-gray coloring and lack of a stem.

Fun Fact

Though the studies are relatively new, it's possible that reishi might soon be billed in mainstream media as the next weapon in the war against obesity. It appears when reishi extracts are consumed with a high-fat diet, the mushroom helps prevent gut inflammation, the proliferation of fatty tissue, and the buildup of harmful bacteria in the bloodstream that can lead to digestion issues and weight gain. Because reishi seems to have the power to alter the ratios of bacteria in the gut, it could help with weight control. But before you mix up a reishi elixir and pull out your skinny jeans, note that the benefits were only seen in people who were very overweight and consuming a diet of very fatty foods. It does not seem that those on relatively healthy, normal diets would yield any significant results. Stay tuned as more research is released.

Chaga [chə-gə]/ *Inonotus obliquus*

USE CHAGA TO

- Ward off the common cold
- Have shiny, thick hair and glowing skin
- Lower inflammation caused by a busy, stressful life

If reishi is the queen of mushrooms, then chaga is the big daddy, the implacable and respected father of the mushroom world. The first recorded usage of chaga dates to seventeenth-century Russia, where it was widely used in folk medicine to cure everything from cancers to gastrointestinal issues. Some historical anecdotes suggest an even longer history. It's believed that Tsar Vladimir Monomakh, who ruled the twelfth-century Kievan Rus', used chaga to cure his lip cancer.

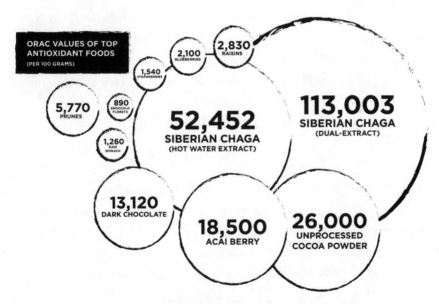

ORAC VALUES OF TOP ANTIOXIDANT FOODS
(PER 100 GRAMS)

1,540 STRAWBERRIES
2,100 BLUEBERRIES
2,830 RAISINS
5,770 PRUNES
890 BROCCOLO FLORETS
1,260 RAW SPINACH
52,452 SIBERIAN CHAGA (HOT WATER EXTRACT)
113,003 SIBERIAN CHAGA (DUAL-EXTRACT)
13,120 DARK CHOCOLATE
18,500 ACAI BERRY
26,000 UNPROCESSED COCOA POWDER

Dual-extracted chaga is one of the highest sources of antioxidants in the world.

Like reishi, chaga has astonishing immunomodulating powers. Chaga's polysaccharides, specifically the beta-glucans, have the ability to boost the production of lymphocytes (a type of white blood cell that regulates the immune response to infectious microorganisms and other foreign substances). Chaga is also one of the single richest sources of antioxidants found in nature, containing an astonishingly wide variety of these cell-protecting compounds. In fact, one dose of dual-extracted chaga (the typical amount found in a single cup of strong chaga tea) packs the same number of antioxidants as thirty pounds of carrots. Why is this important? Antioxidants protect your body from free radicals, also known as oxidants. Overexposure to free radicals leads to cell degeneration, which we experience in the form of chronic fatigue, chronic pain, chronic illness, and cancer. (In Norwegian, chaga is called *kreftkjuke,* which translates to "cancer fungus.")

The triterpenes in chaga also play a major role in shaping its healing properties. One of chaga's most abundant triterpenes is betulin, which has antitumor and anticancer properties. Perhaps more important, though, is that betulin produces a derivative called betulinic acid, which is antibacterial, antiviral, anti-inflammatory, and antioxidant in nature, and has adaptogenic properties. We could point to many specific ailments that

CHAGA IN ACTION

Two of the world's most renowned snowboarders, Terje Håkonsen and Nicolas Müller, use chaga for its anti-inflammatory and skin-protecting abilities. Because these athletes spend so much time with their faces exposed to the sun, high on mountains with little to no shade, chaga acts as an extra, internal layer of sunblock.

the betulinic acid targets and regulates, but that's the beauty of it—it's a nearly infinite list, so it's easier to say that it's essentially a cure for whatever ails you. It's thanks to betulinic acid that chaga can restore balance to your entire system, enabling you to function at your highest potential of health and wellness.

It sounds insane, but chaga *is* sort of insane, as in, insanely good for you. Start by considering its incredible skin-protecting properties. Chaga contains more antioxidant superoxide dismutase (SOD), zinc, and melanin than any other single natural source. You probably know that melanin is responsible for your skin pigmentation, but it's also important for your overall skin health and is a key factor in maintaining healthy eyes and hair. The more melanin you have, the less sensitive your skin is to sun- and windburn, free radicals, solar radiation, and toxins in the air. You'll also have more acute vision and stronger, lusher hair.

For me, chaga has proven itself a health miracle. I travel almost all the time for business, so I am constantly exposed to all different kinds of germs on planes, in taxis, and in hotels, not to mention the countless different toxins that live in the air and vary from location to location. Whenever I feel the inkling of a cold coming on—that scratch that starts in the back of the throat, that sense of body fatigue that has my mind saying "uh-oh"—I double my daily dose of chaga (which is 1,000 to 2,000 milligrams of strong chaga extract in the form of a tea or powder dissolved in liquid). As a result, I have not been sick for a single day in almost a decade. I'm not claiming to be superhuman, but chaga has been remarkably effective at protecting me against the common cold.

Chaga does not have the typical mushroom form of stem and cap but is instead a chunky mass (some call it a *sclerotium* or a *conk*). You can recognize it as a hard, textured, and nearly black "overgrowth" that resembles burnt charcoal. Chaga grows on leafy trees all over the northern hemisphere—primarily on birch trees, though it can be found on ash and maple trees as well. We especially endorse chaga growing on birch trees since it's at least partly thanks to this sacred and powerful tree that chaga absorbs such high concentrations of the good stuff. As further studies are released, it might well be revealed that ash and maple offer unique compounds to render chaga more effective in different ways, but for now, our preference is for birch-grown chaga. Any reputable source should indicate where their chaga originated.

Fun Fact

During World War II, Finns substituted chaga for coffee, as there was a serious scarcity of real coffee but an abundance of chaga growing wild in Finland's forests. Today, it is estimated that between 4 million and 10 million pounds of chaga grow in Finnish woodlands, which may be why some of the foremost chaga researchers in the world are from Finland. Dr. Kirsti Kahlos of the University of Helsinki is a notable example. His team of researchers has conducted multiple studies on the immunomodulating effects of chaga, particularly its potential for use in flu vaccinations and anticancer applications. I'm guessing a lot of chaga coffee is fueling their brains!

Cordyceps [cȯr-di-səps] / Ophiocordyceps sinensis

USE CORDYCEPS TO

- Perform better (both athletically and in the bedroom)
- Increase energy
- Alleviate asthma or bronchitis

Cordyceps is valued primarily for its extraordinary ability to increase energy and reduce fatigue. It's been a centerpiece of traditional Chinese medicine for more than 1,300 years, with the first known record of its use dating back to the Tang Dynasty in AD 620. If historical lore is to be trusted, yak herders in the Himalayas of ancient Tibet and Nepal first noticed the effects of cordyceps when their animals became significantly more frolicky and frisky after grazing in areas where it grew. What those yaks were grazing on is another interesting tidbit: cordyceps's stoma and fruiting body grow out of the mummified carcasses of insect larvae, usually caterpillars—hence its English nickname, the "caterpillar mushroom."

THE INSANE POWER OF FUNGI

Cordyceps is part of the Ascomycetes fungus family, which also includes truffles and morels; *Penicillium*, the mold that naturally produces penicillin; and ergot fungus, the source of the most potent hallucinogen in the world, lysergic acid diethylamide (LSD). The fact that members of the same family can be used in such different manners—as prized culinary mushrooms, or as one of the most prevalent and prescribed antibiotics in the history of Western medicine, or as a powerful mood-altering illegal substance—perfectly illustrates the incredible dichotomy of the fungi kingdom.

In the wild, cordyceps spores inhabit and kill their insect host, stealing all its nutrients to survive. While some strains of cordyceps now grow in other locations (the mountainous regions of Peru, for example), the original celebrated strain of cordyceps grows only on the Himalayan Plateau, at roughly 12,000 feet above sea level, so harvesting them from the wild is both extremely challenging and prohibitively expensive. This in part explains why cordyceps was so valuable in ancient China—it was as rare as it was effective. Today, a Himalayan harvester hopes to find about ten small specimens per day. These treasures may then appear on the shelves of a local apothecary and sell for $500 to $1,300 an ounce—wild cordyceps can cost as much as $20,000 a pound!—meaning that a good harvest year can make a huge difference in the life of the field worker. In fact, some experts estimate that the harvesting of wild cordyceps represents up to 90 percent of the cash income in the areas of Tibet where cordyceps grows, and about 40 percent of all rural area cash income in Tibet. It's a huge business, albeit not a very sustainable one. But don't worry—the cordyceps you will be using in our recipes are almost 100% likely to have been cultivated in a vegan-friendly way through liquid fermentation (the mycelium is strained and dual extracted to create a medicinal deliverable that is as potent as the wild variety).

Cordyceps is most notable for its energizing effects, due to its beta-glucans. Those present in cordyceps, like all other beta-glucans, deliver oxygen to the body on a cellular level, which not only decreases the occurrence of disease but also increases energy and stamina. Cordyceps also significantly boosts adenosine triphosphate (ATP) levels in the body. ATP is the body's main energy supply source and is required for all cellular processes. Cells need energy to activate our muscles and keep us moving. Think of ATP acting on our bodies the way batteries do in a flashlight. When our ATP levels dip, our energy levels take a dive as well. When ATP is recharged, by cordyceps, for example, we shine bright again, moving with ease and alacrity. Because it is so effective at increasing energy and decreasing fatigue, cordyceps is a popular and effective supplement for the elderly who are seeking to counteract the lethargy that often accompanies aging and for athletes who are looking to perform at peak levels. Here's a notable example. Cordyceps first came under the spotlight of mainstream culture in 1993 when China's Olympic women's track-and-field team broke three world records in a single week. The athletes were tested for banned substances and none were detected. Ma Junren, the team's legendary coach, eventually disclosed that the secret to the team's success was a "secret elixir made from the *Cordyceps sinensis* mushroom." Those results are probably a bit more extreme than what you and I will experience, but the fact is that everyone can benefit from using cordyceps as a general rejuvenator, particularly when your body is recovering from illness.

Because of cordyceps's unique ability to boost oxygen flow and increase ATP, it can also have a tremendous impact on respiratory issues, such as asthma or bronchitis. I had a friend who had suffered from asthma since he was a young boy, but as an adult, he started using cordyceps, taking 1,000 to 2,000 milligrams in capsule form daily. After about a month of consistent use, he no longer needed his inhaler or prescription asthma medications.

Cordyceps's anti-inflammatory properties mean that it can help with blood flow, overall heart health, and lowering cholesterol. Its beta-glucans and another chemical compound called cordysepic acid have been known to shrink tumors and directly stimulate lymphocyte production, to kill foreign bodies in the immune system. And then there's the interesting fact that cordyceps has been known to help with libido. This perk is attributed to both the cordysepic acid as well as deoxyadenosine, another chemical acid. Both help with erectile dysfunction by boosting testosterone levels and increasing blood flow by getting things moving in all the right places. Just as it affected those frisky animals in the Himalayas, cordyceps can help out humans in the bedroom. No wonder it's earned the rather unimaginative, yet fitting, nickname "cordysex."

If you happen to be in the Himalayas during a harvest period, you'll recognize Cordyceps by the dark brown "tail" (fruiting body) growing out of the carcasses of dead caterpillars. And if you are there for such an event, be careful, since there is a lot of competition for this highly valued fungi; fights over foraging rights can get ugly. If you're staying put, just use our guide (page 189) to source quality cultivated cordyceps.

Fun Fact

In 2013, cordyceps was at the center of a super-popular video game called *The Last of Us*. Based on actual scientific research, the creators of this survival horror game were inspired by how cordyceps occupies the bodies of the insects it grows from, so they applied the same concept to their virtual humans. In the game, people were taken over by parasitic cordyceps that burrowed into their brains, deriving nutrients from the inside and effectively taking over control of the human body. In real life, there is no way cordyceps could ever burrow into your brain (or any other part of your body), so rest assured that while introducing this mushroom into your life means your energy will surge, your free will will remain intact.

Lion's Mane / *Hericium erinaceus*

USE LION'S MANE TO

- Improve memory
- Boost concentration
- Protect your nervous system

Lion's mane earned its playful moniker because of its unique appearance. Unlike the typical shape of most mushroom fruiting bodies (a smooth cap and stem), lion's mane looks like a cluster of cascading white strands. This waterfall-like "mane" has inspired all kinds of other fun nicknames for the mushroom, including "pom-pom mushroom," "bearded tooth," and "monkey head."

History suggests that lion's mane was used in traditional Chinese medicine specifically for treating stomach and digestive problems, including cancers in these areas of the body. It was also used as a general restorative due to its anti-inflammatory, antibacterial, and immunomodulating properties. But it's lion's mane's effects on the brain that truly distinguish it from other medicinal mushrooms and make it an utterly fascinating subject. It has the ability to repair and regenerate neurons in your body, resulting in improved overall cognitive function, and lion's mane has been known to reverse and mitigate the effects of such neurological diseases such as Parkinson's, Alzheimer's, and dementia, among others.

So how does this all happen? Your body contains nerve growth factor (NGF) proteins, which protect existing neurons and stimulate new neuron growth. These proteins play a crucial role in maintaining the viability of the neurons required for the nervous system to function properly. However, an issue arises when we consider the blood-brain barrier, an internal filtering system whose purpose is to protect the central nervous system by filtering out foreign compounds before they enter the brain. At the same time, the blood-barrier is not permeable by NGF proteins, which are too big to pass through. If your brain is making enough NGF, then all is fine. However, if it's not, the neurons in your brain will not survive and new neurons won't be produced. When the brain doesn't make NGF, it can lead to degenerative neurological diseases such as Parkinson's, Alzheimer's, and dementia.

Amazingly, lion's mane stimulates the synthesis of NGF. How? Let's go back to its Latin name, *Hericium erinaceus*. *Hericenones* are the molecular compounds that stimulate the brain to make more NGF. *Erinacines* are even more powerful compounds that are small enough to permeate the blood-brain barrier. Together, these compounds can foster NGF production from *within* the brain. It's pretty astonishing. Lion's mane not only has the potential to help those suffering from neurological disorders, but through NGF stimulation, it can potentially reverse the cognitive deterioration that creeps up on all of us as we age. And unlike most medicines used for cognitive function—prescribed or holistic—there are no known side effects to lion's mane. It can be taken every day (in capsule form or as a powder dissolved in liquid—see dosage chart, page 37) without risk of adverse consequences.

Aside from lion's mane's incredible medicinal properties, it's also truly delicious on its own. It does not need to be extracted or processed into a powder before use—you can simply sauté it in butter and enjoy. When eaten in its whole form, its medicinal potency is not as concentrated as when it's consumed as an extract, but you'll still reap many great benefits. Because of its meaty texture, it's long been a popular meat replacement in Asian dishes. You'll find you can easily sneak it into many dishes, even desserts, for an added brain boost (we'll show you how on pages 144 through 149)!

I became fully convinced of lion's mane's neurological effects after a good friend of mine was injured in a surfing accident a few years ago. A crashing surfboard hit her hard, and she incurred some brain damage as a result. She could still function, but the accident damaged the nerves in her brain to the point where she often lost focus and had frequent dizzy spells. She started taking 1,500 to 3,000 milligrams of lion's mane daily, and after six to eight weeks, her dizzy spells were far less frequent and she was able to focus better and for longer periods of time. Though she is not cured, her condition has improved steadily since then, something she readily attributes to her use of lion's mane.

You can identify lion's mane by its puffy mane of cascading white strands. While no other mushroom has quite the same do, bear's head and comb tooth can look somewhat similar. Lion's mane grows out of dead and decaying hardwood trees all over the world, but is particularly prevalent across North America, China, Japan, and Europe.

Fun Fact

The discovery of NGF proteins is credited to Italian scientist Rita Levi-Montalcini, and earned her (and her colleague Stanley Cohen) the 1986 Nobel Prize in Physiology and Medicine. The first Nobel laureate to live for more than one hundred years, Rita died at age 103, and it's believed she used NGF eye drops daily. She credited her longevity and the intellectual acumen she maintained right up until the time of her death to these drops. Since lion's mane is the most abundant natural source of NGF proteins, there's no need for you to use eye drops if you introduce the mushroom into your regimen. Bonus: You'll be getting a host of other benefits that Levi-Montalcini's drops did not have, so imagine how long you could live!

Shiitake [shē-təh-kē] / *Lentinula edodes*

USE SHIITAKE TO

- Have clear, glowing skin
- Support your liver
- Lower cholesterol

Shiitake is one of the most widely cultivated mushrooms in the world, second only to the button mushroom, making it the most easily accessible medicinal mushroom. A veritable culinary delicacy featured in Asian cooking for centuries, shiitake has become increasingly popular in American cooking over the past decade. Delicious when used fresh, dried shiitake is also a favorite among chefs and home cooks who are seeking a more concentrated flavor. For strictly medicinal purposes, shiitake can be taken as a supplement in capsule form or as an extract. Each preparation will deliver a host of benefits and how you decide to consume it will vary depending on your particular needs.

Medicinal use of shiitake dates back at least as far as AD 100 in China, when it was used to treat and prevent upper respiratory diseases, boost circulation, increase energy, decrease fatigue, and as a general "chi"-enhancing elixir. It comes as little surprise that it was also used to combat and prevent signs of aging.

Today, we know shiitake to be a truly rare superfood, as it contains seven of the nine essential amino acids (amino acids are the building blocks of proteins that must be consumed from outside sources, as the human body does not produce them). Shiitake also contains a host of essential enzymes (like amylase and cellulase, both of which aid in digestion), is a good source of vital minerals (including magnesium and potassium, which have antioxidant properties), and essential vitamins (such as B and D—see our Fun Fact).

Shiitake's major health benefits are its immunomodulating abilities and its impact on the cardiovascular system. Regarding the immune system, one of the polysaccharides in shiitakes is lentinan, which stimulates and activates the different varieties of white blood cells that fight off infections. Lentinan has been especially powerful in combatting the effects of HIV and liver disease, making it an effective treatment for any sort of bodily detoxification. Perhaps surprisingly, this can even include improved skin appearance. People don't often connect chronic acne or persistent breakouts with what's going on with our internal organs, but our skin is really a mirror for whatever is happening in our liver. A fully functioning liver often equates to a flawless face.

Shiitake can also have tremendous effects on the cardiovascular system, as it can prevent substances from binding to the linings of blood vessels. For example, eritadenine, one of shiitake's bioactive compounds, has repeatedly shown to help lower cholesterol by inhibiting its absorption in the bloodstream. It does this in part by suppressing the accumulation of lipids in the liver tissue and helping to eliminate cholesterol through the blood vessels, rather than allowing fatty acids to build up. Along with numerous anti-inflammatory and antiviral capacities, shiitake's ability to improve blood circulation could mean much for those suffering from rheumatoid arthritis. To that end, shiitake's effects are continuing to be more seriously studied.

SHIITAKE IN ACTION

A powerful story showcasing shiitake's healing properties involves a young teenage celebrity I know who was quietly suffering from a particularly pervasive and tenacious case of acne. Though he was using aggressive treatments, his skin was increasingly becoming a source of stress on his professional life as a public figure. The young man started taking 1,500 milligrams of shiitake extract, stopped taking his prescription, and in about a month his skin had cleared considerably, improving until the acne was completely gone.

You can identify shiitake by its medium-size, umbrella-shaped brown cap. The edges of the cap roll inward and the underside and stem of the mushroom are white. In the wild, shiitake grows on hardwood trees primarily in the mountainous regions of China, Japan, Indonesia, and Taiwan. Commercially, shiitake is commonly grown in sawdust and grain (logs are more expensive, heavier, and can be harder to obtain). Log-grown shiitake is more potent than sawdust-grown, so this is another reason to do your research when sourcing mushrooms. If your vendor does not cite where their shiitake grew, it was most likely grown in sawdust or grain.

Fun Fact

Many chefs prefer to use sun-dried shiitake, as the drying enhances the mushroom's flavor. As an added bonus, the sun's ultraviolet rays convert ergosterol (a derivative of a triterpene sterol found in shiitake and other fungi) into vitamin D_2. With up to a hundredfold increase in vitamin D, sun-dried shiitakes can be a significant dietary source of your requirement of the vitamin. Because of the media hype a few years ago surrounding widespread vitamin D deficiencies in the United States, many companies capitalized on the moneymaking potential, and the vitamin D supplement market was quickly saturated. Be wary of these supplements, as many of them are questionable. Shiitake, on the other hand, directly delivers pure vitamin D.

Maitake [mā-tək-ē] / *Grifola frondosa*

USE MAITAKE TO

- Manage weight naturally
- Stabilize blood sugar
- Improve digestion

In Japanese, *maitake* means "dancing mushroom," a name that historical lore suggests was derived from the Samurai. Foraging for these precious mushrooms often involved long and strenuous escapades deep in the mountains and forests of Japan, and it is believed that the Samurai danced for joy upon discovering these edible treasures. Other names by which you might recognize this superfood include "sheep's head" and "ram's head."

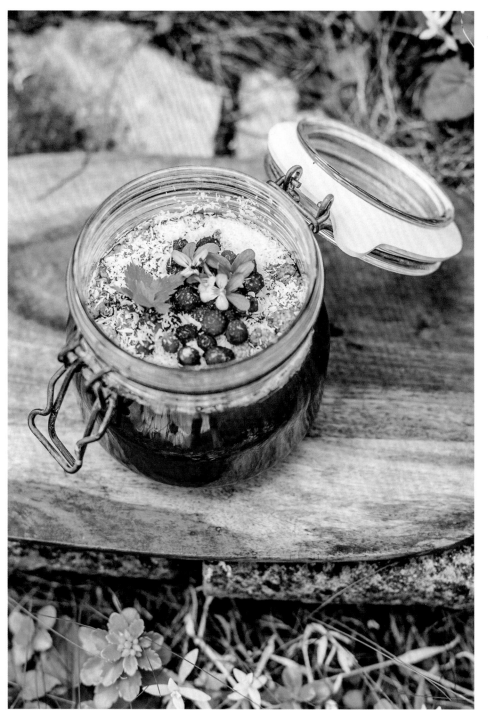

Chaga Jelly Bowl
(page 120)

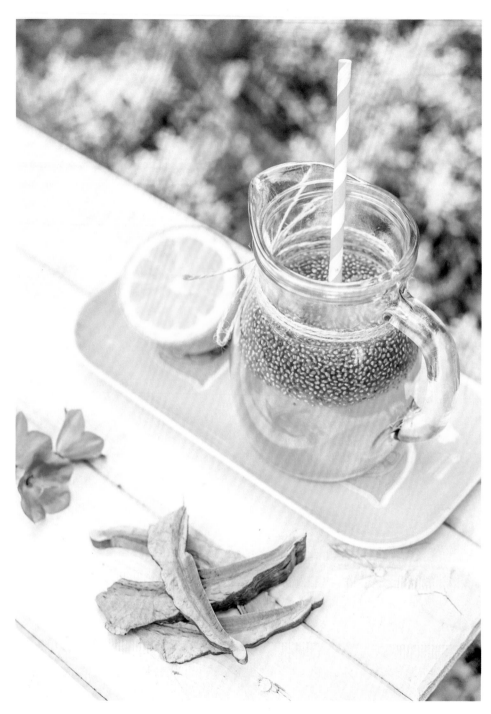

Reishi-Mucuna Lemonade

(page 150)

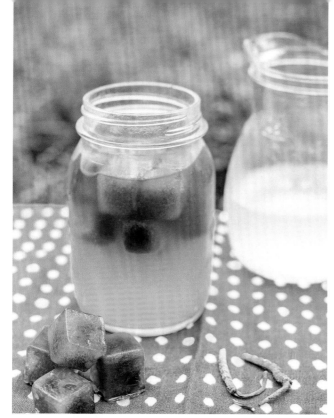

Cordyceps Cubes
with Coconut Water
(page 138)

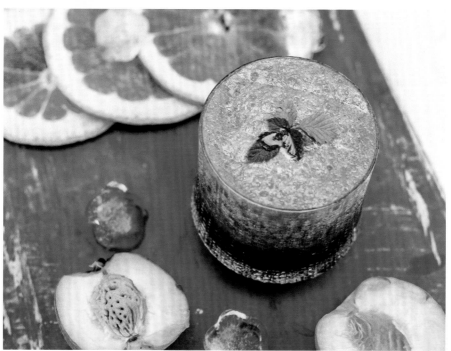

Cordysex on the Beach
(page 174)

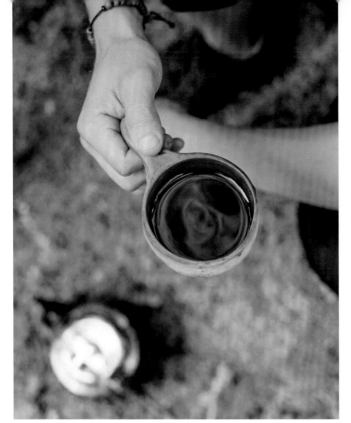

Chaga Un-Coffee
(page 154)

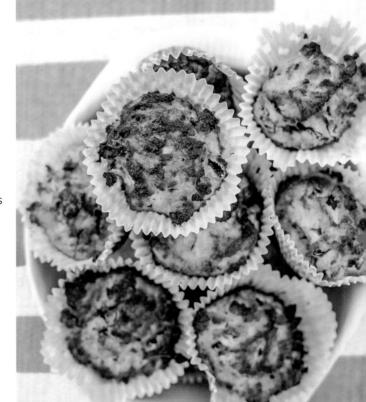

Maitake Muffins
(page 84)

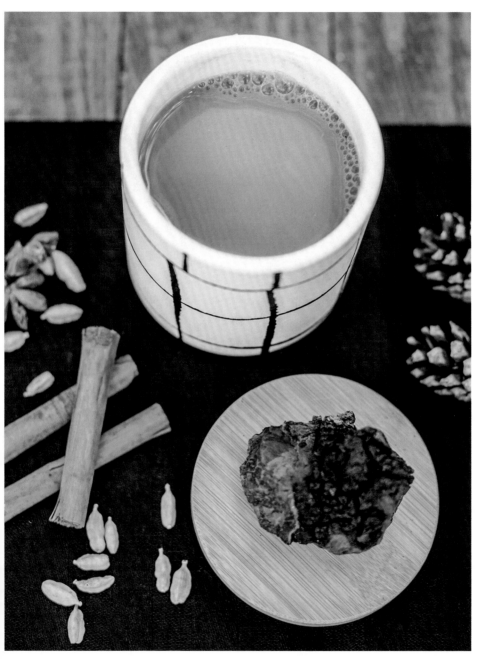

Chaga Chai

(page 88)

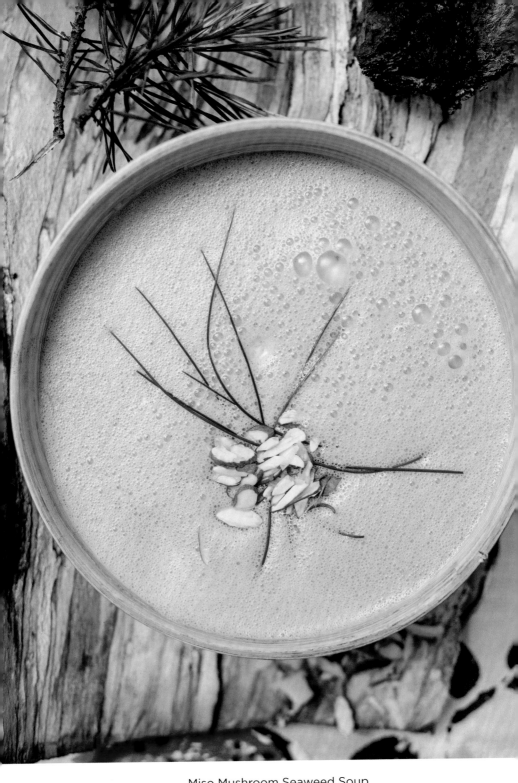

Miso Mushroom Seaweed Soup

(page 98)

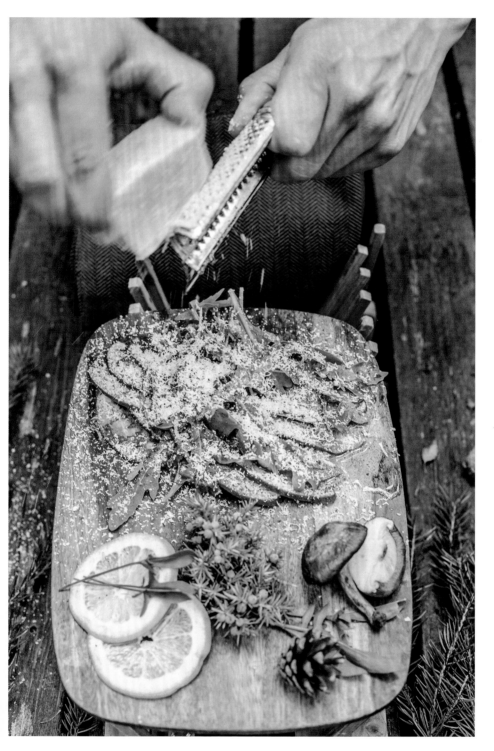

Shiitake Carpaccio

(page 83)

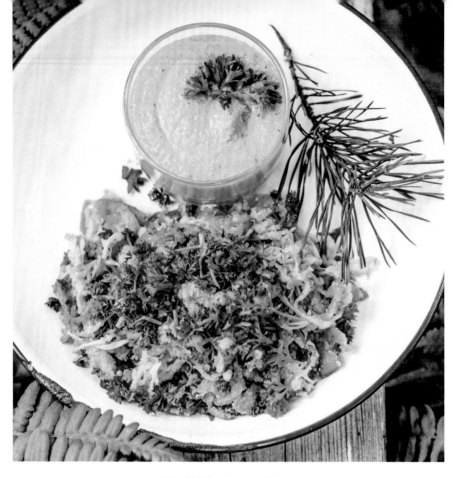

Enoki Mushroom Fries
(page 180)

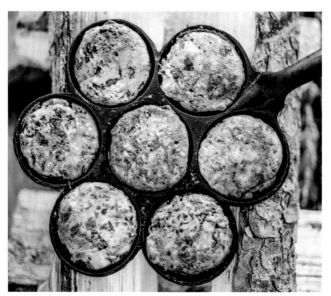

Lion's Mane
Pancakes
(page 146)

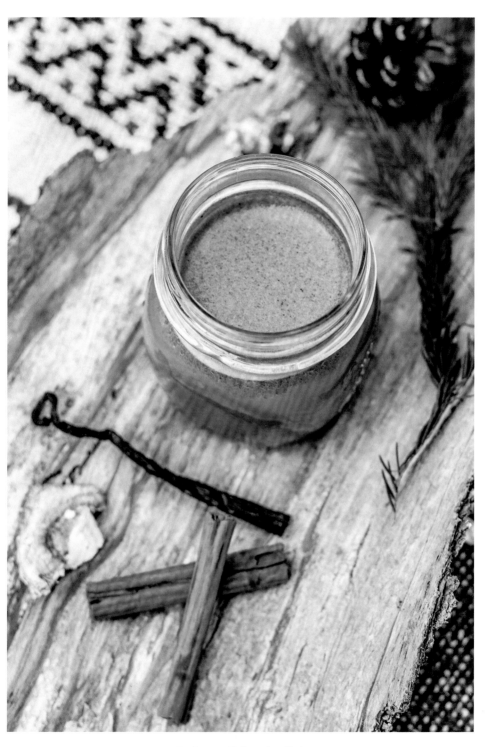

Turkey Tail Carob Elixir

(page 110)

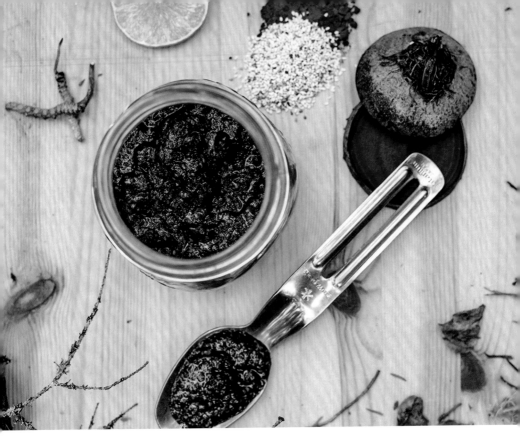

Superfood Sports Gel with Cordyceps and Beets

(page 141)

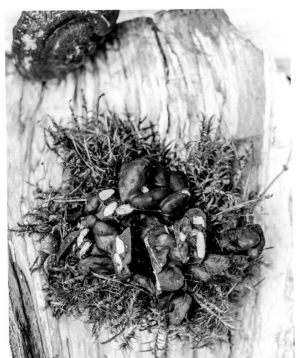

Reishi Chocolate Almonds

(page 112)

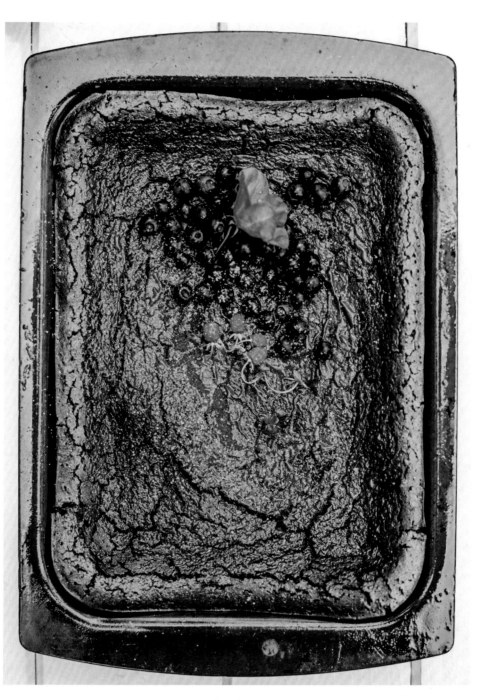

Superfood Mudcake

(page 166)

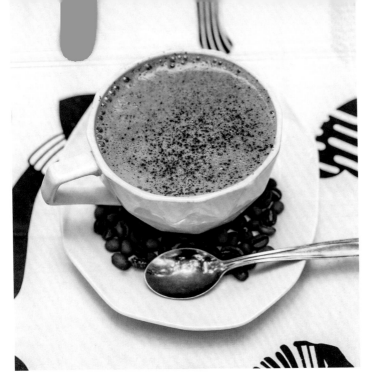

Reishi Cappuccino
(page 159)

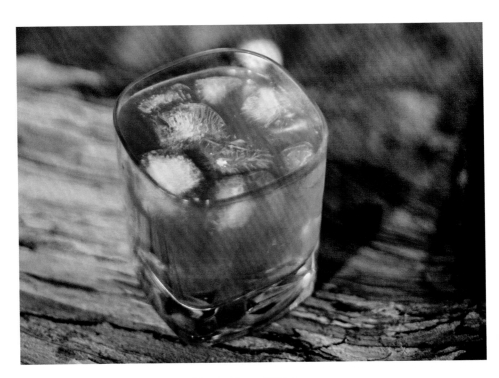

Lion's Mane Whiskey
(page 178)

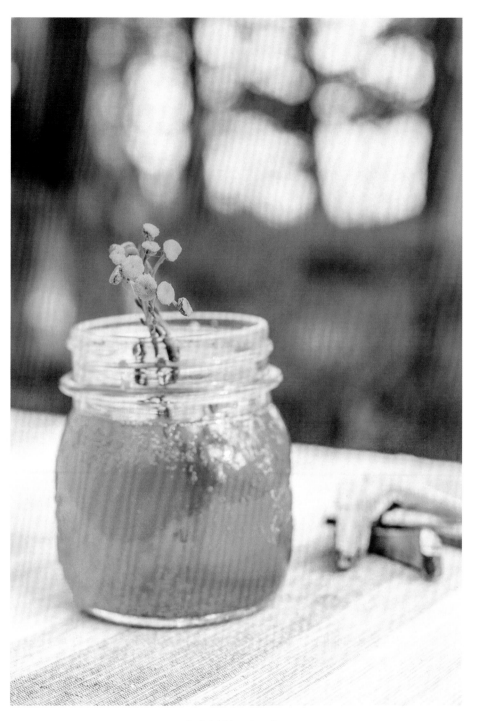

Reishi Kombucha
(page 103)

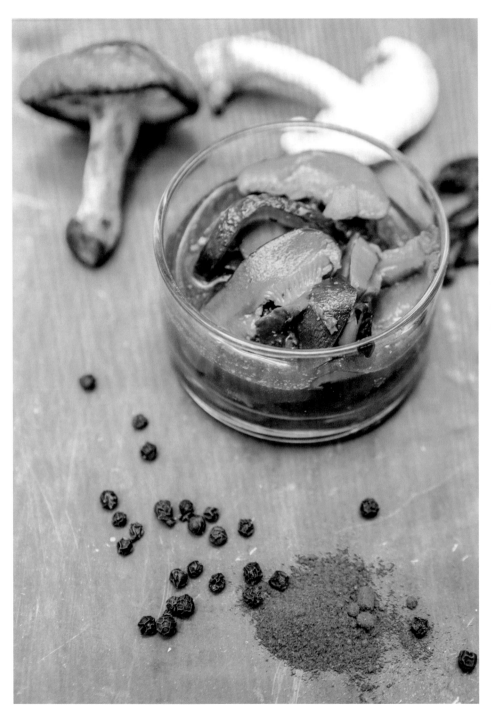

Pickled and Dehydrated Shiitake Jerky

(page 92)

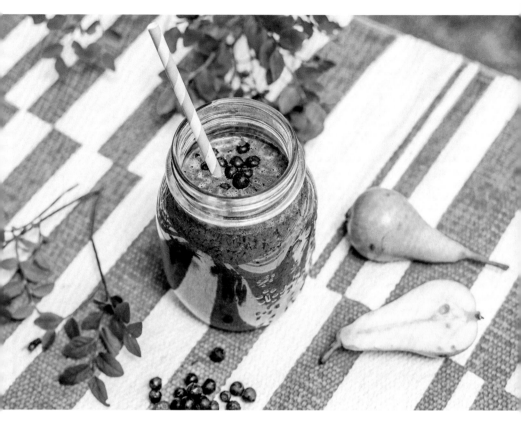

Berry Blast Smoothie
(page 130)

Chaga Skin Cream
(page 128)

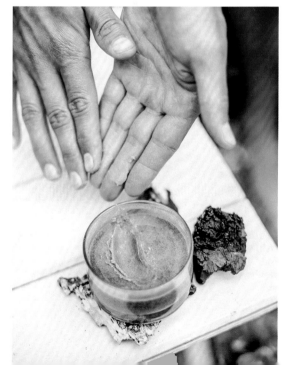

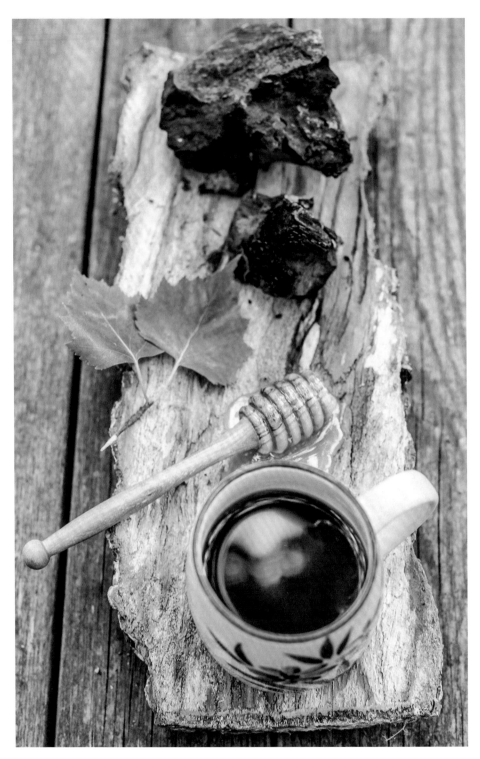

Chaga Decoction, aka 'Shroom Tea

(page 74)

Like many of our other top ten medicinal mushrooms, maitake has powerful immunomodulating properties, particularly due to its beta-glucan polysaccharides. What separates maitake from other medicinal mushrooms is its SX-fraction, a water-soluble compound so named because of its ability to counteract the effects of Syndrome X. Also known as metabolic syndrome, Syndrome X is not one disease, per se, but rather refers to a group of risk factors, including high blood sugar, high cholesterol, high blood pressure, and excess fat, that feed on one another to negatively impact your health and wellness. The SX-fraction compound has the potential to reduce blood glucose levels, blood pressure, and body weight, so it can potentially work wonders on those suffering from diabetes or obesity. SX-fraction also works as an adaptogen, meaning it will not only benefit those who are hyperglycemic but can also stabilize blood sugar levels in those who are hypoglycemic. As with many health issues, solving the root of the problem often creates a positive domino effect on overall health and wellness. In the case of diabetes, if blood sugar is regulated and insulin resistance eliminated, it's possible that kidney and renal functions, which often deteriorate as a result of diabetes, could be stabilized and any existing damage potentially reversed. Crazy stuff, isn't it?

MAITAKE IN ACTION

A woman I worked with years ago suffered from intestinal candidiasis (a yeastlike bad fungus that had accumulated in her GI tract due to a bacterial imbalance in her body). Because candida is a strain of yeast, she was sure she could not eat mush-

(continued)

rooms for fear of literally feeding the problem. However, it's a myth that those suffering from candida cannot eat mushrooms—in fact, many medicinal mushrooms like maitake and reishi have antifungal properties that work to eliminate bad fungi such as candida. Once she realized that mushrooms could actually help her, she started taking 3,000 milligrams of maitake extract daily, and within a few months, her candida had disappeared completely and her digestive system was back to normal.

You can identify maitake by its clusterlike form that resembles the feathers of a fluffed chicken—hence the popular name for the mushroom in the United States, "hen-of-the-woods." Maitake primarily grows at the base of oak or elm trees in the northeastern parts of Japan and North America. Maitake can be eaten fresh or dried and is a popular culinary mushroom used by chefs the world over. It's also often taken in powder form after an extraction process.

Fun Fact

If you're searching for flavor, look no further than maitake. It contains l-glutamate, the amino acid responsible for that much-touted and oft-elusive "umami" taste. Known as the "fifth flavor," you can experience umami by eating bacon, Parmesan cheese, and foods containing the artificial flavor-enhancer monosodium glutamate (MSG). None of these options are nearly as healthy as maitake, though, so look to mushrooms for your next culinary high.

Turkey Tail / *Coriolus versicolor* or *Trametes versicolor*

USE TURKEY TAIL TO

- Treat the common cold and flu
- Aid digestion
- Help heal infections

Turkey tail earned its name due to the mushroom's fan shape, which resembles the tail end of fall's favorite bird. Its Latin name means "of several colors," which is also fitting as this mushroom can be identified by the concentric circles of varying colors that appear on its fruiting body. A pervasive grower, turkey tail is the easiest to forage of all the medicinal mushrooms simply because of its ubiquity—you can find it almost anywhere, growing on dead or fallen hardwood trees, stumps, or branches. This quality may have been what led to its use in traditional Chinese medicine—it has been said that ancient Taoists were astonished by how easily this colorful mushroom grew on pine, which was a notoriously antifungal tree. They concluded that a mushroom of such tenacity and strength must contain incredible medicinal properties.

And so it does. Like many other medicinal mushrooms, turkey tail is full of polysaccharides and triterpenes that give it its immunomodulating properties, providing overall immune support and regulation to put you on the path to your healthiest self. What sets turkey tail apart from the rest of the medicinal mushrooms are two of its unique beta-glucans: polysaccharide krestin (PSK) and polysaccharide peptide (PSP).

PSK has received national media attention for its anticancer properties. In Western medicine, the goal of cancer treatments such as chemotherapy and radiation is to kill the cancer cells, but a serious consequence of these aggressive treatments is that the immune system is often left compromised—you cannot kill all the bad cells without also taking out many of the good. What is amazing about the PSK and PSP in turkey tail is that they have the ability to regenerate white blood cells (which are necessary to ward off infection) and stimulate the activity and creation of T-cells, macrophages, and natural killer (NK) cells, enabling the immune system to once again ward off and destroy pathogens. As of this printing, PSK has been more thoroughly studied than PSP, particularly in Japan, where, as early as the 1980s, the government allowed PSK to be used to treat several types of cancer. Today, it is the best-selling anticancer drug on the Japanese market and is used in combination with surgery, chemotherapy, and radiation therapy. Though PSP is a newer discovery, research suggests that it's significantly more powerful than PSK, which is an exciting notion for developing future cancer treatments. Turkey tail has also proven successful in stimulating the regeneration of bone marrow damaged by cancer treatments and has also been effective in treating human papillomavirus (HPV) and hepatitis C.

TURKEY TAIL IN ACTION

What drove turkey tail's seriously healing potential home for me was a TED Talk given by world-renowned mycologist Paul Stamets, in which he brought turkey tail to the attention of the masses by sharing a personal tale involving his mother. At age eighty-four, she had been diagnosed with the second most aggressive case of stage 4 breast cancer a doctor at the Swedish Cancer Institute in Seattle, Washington, had seen in more than twenty years of practice. The doctor suggested she try turkey tail in conjunction with her treatment, as it was being clinically tried at the time (ironically, Stamets was supplying the turkey tail to the medical study). His mother started taking eight capsules of turkey tail each day and during this 2011 TED Talk, just two years after his mother was diagnosed and given mere months to live, Mrs. Stamets came to the stage, weeping with her son as they announced that she was completely cancer-free.

You can identify turkey tail by its fanlike shape; it often grows in tiered clusters on dead or fallen hardwood trees. The multicolored concentric bands are usually in shades of brown, black, and deep red, but can be blue and green as well. The mushroom has a thick, leathery feel; is stemless; and has small pores on its underside instead of gills like on many other mushrooms.

Fun Fact

Foraging 101 is all about turkey tail, because if there is one mushroom you can find on your lunch break, it's this one. Once you find it, you'll start seeing it everywhere—seriously. Note that turkey tail is not edible in its natural form, so don't immediately try to gobble up your woodsy finds. The most common ways to consume it are in powdered and liquid extract forms (see page 192 for sources).

Enoki [ē-nō-kē] / *Flammulina velutipes*

USE ENOKI TO

- Improve skin quality/look younger
- Optimize immune function
- Help with joint pains

While used in traditional Chinese medicine, enoki's versatility in the culinary realm, where it has long been a celebrated staple in Asian cuisine, is what distinguishes it from many other mushrooms. That, and that it's also one of the most visually appealing mushrooms, with its unique, delicate shape. Enoki grows in clusters of slender, pure white stalks, each capped by a tiny round head, which has earned it nicknames like "velvet foot," "snow puff mushroom," and "winter mushroom." Enoki's full name is actually enokitake (*take* in Japanese translates to "mushroom"), but the name has all but officially been shortened to enoki (meaning "hackberry" in Japanese), which is the name of the tree the mushroom often grows on. In fact, enoki mushrooms growing in the wild on hackberry and other hardwood trees do not grow nearly as white as the ones we see at grocers and farmers' markets—these are typically cultivated indoors, as the supply needed to meet their high culinary demand often surpasses what can be foraged. This lack of sunlight during cultivation results in the pure, snowy white enoki we've come to know.

Its mild, delicious flavor and elegant appearance aside, enoki is a powerful medicinal mushroom thanks to the many antioxidants it contains. One antioxidant in particular, ergothioneine, not only rids the body of free radicals but has proven to be especially powerful in reducing photodamage on the skin. As a result, you'll find enoki in many antiaging skin products. Because ergothioneine creates intercellular stimulation to produce ATP, enoki also has myriad possibilities as an anticancer agent, with particularly fruitful studies showing positive effects in treating lymphoma and prostate cancer. Proflanin and flammulin, two of enoki's polysaccharides, have also been shown to have tremendous effects on boosting immunity and eliminating cancerous cells. Because of Proflanin's unusually high protein to carbohydrate ratio (10:1) it's much lighter than many of the beta-glucans found in other medicinal mushrooms. This just means it works faster and more efficiently at targeting foreign pathogens. Flammulin has its own special properties and has been especially effective in fighting melanoma. Additionally, lectin, a protein that naturally occurs in enoki, enhances the production of its antioxidants, making this mushroom an antiviral, antibacterial, and overall restorative immunoregulator for achieving optimal wellness both inside and out.

This white beauty also contains high levels of vitamin B_3. In fact, 1 cup of raw enoki contains 23 percent of the vitamin B_3 we require daily. The anti-inflammatory properties of niacinamide, a specific type of vitamin B_3 found in enoki, can alleviate joint pain and stiffness, and provide arthritis relief. Enoki also has twice as much fiber as cabbage, so it's effective at managing blood sugar and aiding digestion. And it contains the minerals thiamine, folate, and riboflavin, making it a good supplement for those in need of thyroid support.

You can find enoki growing in clusters on dead hardwood trees in cooler temperatures from late fall into winter. Remember that wild enoki is not the pure white mushroom we are used to seeing on store shelves—rather, they are dark orange to brown in color with a sticky-to-the-touch cap. While wild enoki mushrooms are probably a bit better for our health, cultivated enoki still holds significant medicinal value.

Fun Fact

Dr. Tetsuro Ikewawa, a former epidemiologist at the Research Institute of the National Cancer Center in Tokyo, performed a study after noting that the incidence of cancer in Nagano was significantly lower than that of the immediately surrounding areas. He soon learned that Nagano was the epicenter of enoki mushroom growth and that enoki cultivators and farmers, along with their families, had the lowest incidence of cancer of all. This group was nearly immune to developing cancer, presumably because they were consuming more enoki than anyone else—someone had to eat up the less-than-perfect specimens that vendors and retailers refused to buy!

Oyster Mushroom / *Pleurotus ostreatus* or *Pleurotus populinus*

USE OYSTER MUSHROOMS TO

- Relax and improve your mood
- Improve skin quality/look younger
- Lower your cholesterol

Like shiitake and maitake, the oyster mushroom is a veritable culinary delicacy, and has historically been used in Asian cuisines as a meat substitute due to its high levels of protein and meaty texture (though it's perfectly edible and delicious, this mushroom *must* be cooked before eating as the heat eliminates a toxic protein it contains). Oyster mushrooms are also known as "tree oyster," "oyster shelf," and "hiratake," which means "flat mushroom" in Japanese. These nicknames are indicative of the oyster mushroom's flat-tiered clustered growth pattern.

Oyster mushrooms also contain powerful beta-glucans with tremendous immunomodulating powers, and they have proven especially effective in combating colon and breast cancers. Oyster mushrooms also contain lovastatin, a naturally occurring chemical that lowers cholesterol levels. Aside from its ability to reduce cholesterol, act as an anticancer agent, and serves as a delicious meat substitute, the oyster mushroom also contains high levels of zinc and iron and plenty of B vitamins. In particular, it contains vitamin B_6, which works wonders to calm the body and boost spirits (B_6 stimulates the body to produce serotonin, a neurotransmitter that regulates our sleep and mood). For this reason, we often like to suggest eating oyster mushrooms in the evening, as its mellowing properties can melt away the stress of the workday instead of a glass of wine

OYSTER MUSHROOM

In addition to being medical marvels, oyster mushrooms hold significant environmental potential. This mushroom has the ability to break down hydrocarbon molecules—which are present in toxins and contaminants such as diesel fuel, gasoline, oil, plastics, and polychlorinated biphenyls (PCBs were used in coolants and insulation materials, among other things, before they were banned in the United States during the late 1970s). When oyster mushroom mycelium is scattered over polluted areas, the mycelium absorbs and breaks down the chemicals, outgases the pollutants, and purifies the contaminated soil. It goes without saying that you would not want to eat the mushrooms that sprout from these areas, but think about the impact these mushrooms can have on oil spills—we can seriously save the planet, one fungus at a time.

(or with it, if it's been a really tough day). Put your feet up while you're at it, too—in traditional Chinese medicine, oyster mushrooms were often used for joint and muscle relaxation.

You can identify oyster mushrooms by their flat-tiered growth pattern of whitish clusters. They have gills on the underside of the caps and a barely discernible stem, and they grow in warm and temperate climates on Aspen trees. Note that there are many mushrooms in the *Pleurotus* family, so it's pretty easy to accidentally pick a different mushroom (even with all my foraging experience, I've definitely done that a number of times). It's highly unlikely that what you mistake for an oyster mushroom would be poisonous, but it probably would not have the same medicinal properties or flavor as the real deal.

Fun Fact

If you're looking to fade freckles and sun spots, forget lemon juice and turn to oyster mushrooms instead. They contain kojicacid, a natural skin lightener, so taking high doses (see the dosage chart on page 37) of oyster mushroom extract daily should allow you to say farewell to freckles in a few months or even weeks.

Mushroom Trivia Tidbit

Want to grow your own oyster mushrooms? This mushroom is one of the easiest in the kingdom to cultivate, so go on and become a fungi farmer by purchasing a growing starter kit (we like the ones from Back to the Roots and Fungi Perfecti). Bonus: It's a way-fun activity for kids.

Tremella [trē-məl-ə] / *Tremella fuciformis*

* Improve skin quality/look younger
* Protect your body against pathogens
* Alleviate asthma or chest congestion

Tremella is another medicinal mushroom with a wonderfully distinct appearance. It's a member of the jelly fungus family and has a unique gelatinous texture. Its wobbly structure has earned it the nicknames "yellow brain," "golden jelly fungus," "yellow trembler," and "witch's butter." Tremella closely resembles a loofah shower sponge, which is a fitting comparison because one of the main reasons we admire tremella is for its power as a "beauty mushroom"; it plays an astounding role in reversing and counteracting the aging process.

In traditional Chinese medicine, tremella was valued as an antiaging ingredient. One of tremella's polysaccharides has remarkable water retention properties—it can hold up to five hundred times its weight in water, much more than both hyaluronic acid and glycerin, two ingredients commonly used in expensive "rejuvenating" and moisturizing skin products—and is the primary reason tremella can help restore a youthful appearance to the skin. When applied topically (such as in a skin cream where tremella extract powder has been combined with oils like shea butter or coconut oil), tremella not only enhances the skin by making it soft and supple but also stimulates the production of superoxide dismutase (SOD), a naturally occurring enzyme in the dermis and epidermis. As you might recall from the chaga section, SOD is an antioxidant that protects the skin from free radicals. By stimulating SOD production, tremella acts as a protective and regenerative anti-inflammatory for the skin. And like oyster mushrooms, tremella also contains kojic acid, which can help fade freckles and lighten dark spots.

Tremella was also used in cough syrups in traditional Chinese medicine as a way to treat chest congestion and asthma. Its hydrating qualities help replenish bodily fluids, making it a coveted remedy for many illnesses. This fungus has all the immuno-modulatory effects we've come to expect from medicinal mushrooms and also has the potential to regulate blood sugar and lower cholesterol. Tremella has also been effective in regenerating bone marrow destroyed or damaged through radiation treatments by restoring the blood-producing mechanism to the bone marrow, contains more vitamin D than any other known single food source, is loaded with antioxidants, and has vast amounts of fiber.

Though it's an edible mushroom, tremella does not taste much like anything, which makes it easy to sneak into a variety of dishes. Its gelatinous texture makes it a natural choice for use in desserts, and it's often used in Asian dishes like *lok mei*, the Chinese equivalent of chicken noodle soup.

TREMELLA IN ACTION

I can vouch for tremella's reputation as a beauty mushroom, as I've seen firsthand the incredible glow it creates. My good friend has been modeling for more than ten years, a feat in itself, as modeling is typically a short career. She attributes her perfect complexion to regular use of medicinal mushrooms—tremella being her favorite—and an infrared sauna (an incredible health and wellness tool that heats the body from the inside out to eliminate toxins). At photo shoots, makeup artists have marveled that her glowing skin requires far less makeup than that of models who are at least ten years her junior. This is great news for all of us—we can have flawless skin, too, with no aggressive skin regimens, expensive potions, or juice cleansing required.

You can find tremella growing on hardwood trees all over Europe, in parts of the United States (Northern California in particular), and the mountains of Taiwan. The white-to-yellow wobbly cluster will make you do a double-take: Is that a jellyfish that sprouted in the woods?

Fun Fact

It is said that Yan Guifei, one of the four beauties of ancient China and the favorite concubine of Tang Emperor Xuanzong (685–762 BC), used tremella regularly to achieve what was referred as a "face that put flowers to shame." Perhaps it was her glowing complexion, courtesy of tremella's hydrating and restorative effects, that so enamored the powerful ruler and resulted in Guifei earning high appointments and positions for her family members.

AFTER MEETING THESE TEN MUSHROOMS and learning just the tip of the iceberg in terms of their potential as health powerhouses, you're probably perplexed as to why more people aren't using fungi to cure diseases, ward off illnesses, eliminate toxins and pollutants, achieve youthful radiance, and generally function at optimal levels of wellness. It's possible that it's because the fungi kingdom's vast potential has only received minimal exposure in mainstream media because pharmaceutical companies cannot profit from natural remedies, since they are not patentable. But the good news is that we have loads more information now, and we're using it to be the healthiest, best looking, most harmonious versions of ourselves that we can be. We want that for you, too, and that's why we've introduced you to these ten mushrooms—so we can all be funguys. Now let's eat!

4

MUSHROOM MAGIC IN THE KITCHEN

n this chapter, we've included fifty mushroom recipes, what we think are the best of the best. We've selected these dishes for their effectiveness with regards to health and wellness, ease of preparation, and—this goes without saying—deliciousness. We also chose these because we want to inspire you with some surprising ways to use mushrooms. Sure, a classic mushroom risotto is always a welcome sight on the table, and we've included one here for that reason—but you won't find too many more expected dishes like that. Instead, we've included recipes that will quickly take you from "Wait, really?" to "Yes, really!"

Because you may be looking to alleviate particular ailments or address specific medical concerns, we have divided the recipes into categories based on today's most prevalent health issues, many of which affect us all to some degree. However, just because a recipe is included as a way to help with, say, hormonal balance, doesn't preclude it from also being very effective against inflammation. The beauty of these recipes, as is the case with all medicinal and culinary mushrooms, is that none are mere one-hit wonders; they will all have multiple positive effects on your overall health and wellness.

So head to the kitchen—it's time to cook up some mushroom magic.

Pantry and Preparation Guide

A few important things to note as you prepare to cook:

1. Be sure to check out our Shopping Guide (page 189) for tips, resources, and guidance in terms of sourcing quality products. Many of the recipes included in this section call for mushrooms in extract or powder form. While these items may not be stocked at all specialty grocers or natural food stores, you can certainly purchase them online. Our guide will direct you to the most reputable sites for doing so. If you are feeling ambitious, visit us online (foursigmatic.com) for a step-by-step tutorial on making your own mushroom extracts and powders.

2. Special kitchen equipment is not required, though you will need a blender and a food processor for some recipes. We find that a Vitamix or other high-powered blender can make a big difference in terms of the consistency of the finished product, but a standard blender or food processor will work just fine, too. An espresso machine is helpful for the coffee drinks, but not essential. And should you find yourself getting really into fermenting, you might want to look into more specialized equipment down the road.

3. We're all about using ingredients that provide the maximum health benefits. When it comes to ingredients like chocolate, oils, or butter, use the best quality you can find and afford. Though usually more expensive, options that have minimal additives and fillers will make a big difference in flavor and texture. You can find other specialty, nonmushroom ingredients like tocotrienols, cacao butter, coconut flour, coconut butter, mucuna, maca, and more at most natural food stores, even Whole Foods. They can also be purchased online from Amazon, Thrive Market, and other webstores. Be sure to do your research and purchase from a reputable source.

Chaga Decoction, aka 'Shroom Tea

Paleo • Vegan • Gluten-free • Low-glycemic • Low-fat

Apples are great and all, but it's a cup of this chaga goodness a day that really keeps the doctor away. We've opted not to delineate it as beneficial for any single ailment because it helps with *every* ailment. It's a daily tonic that can lead to incredible overall wellness. Regular consumption of chaga will support and regulate the immune system, alleviate digestive issues, boost the production of cancer-fighting cells, and leave you with radiant skin, lush hair, and more acute vision.

Coffee lovers will be pleased to hear that although we've dubbed this drink a mushroom *tea*, its bitter flavor is actually quite similar to that of coffee. It's a great anytime drink because you can customize the flavor—try adding vanilla, anise, ginger, or different spices and fruits—based on the season and your mood.

SERVES 4

TOTAL TIME: 12 TO 24 HOURS

> 1 tablespoon ground chaga (see Notes)
>
> Spices, fruits, and herbs such as licorice root, vanilla bean, star anise, slices of ginger, fresh mint, or berries (optional)
>
> Nut milk of choice (optional)
>
> Agave, raw honey, or stevia (optional)

1. In a medium saucepan, combine the chaga and 3¾ cups water and bring to a rolling boil over high heat. Once the water is boiling, reduce the heat to maintain a simmer.
2. Simmer the chaga brew, uncovered, for 12 to 24 hours (see Notes), stirring every hour or so.

3. For additional flavor, add the flavorings of your choice during the last 30 minutes of boiling (regardless of how long you are brewing the tea).

4. Strain the tea into mugs. Enjoy as is or doctor it up with nut milk and natural sweetener to your liking. Due to the high quantity of antioxidants the tea contains, extra can be stored in an airtight container in the refrigerator and reheated for up to 5 days. However, we advocate for potency and recommend drinking it within 1 to 2 days to reap the most benefits.

Notes • *Grinding chaga is harder than it sounds. It's easiest to buy it preground (see our Shopping Guide, page 189), but if you decide to do it yourself, just know that many knives, Microplane graters, and blenders have been damaged in the process. Dry chaga can be chopped into smaller pieces, while cooked chaga will break up a little more easily. Once it's ground, the chaga will keep for years provided it is kept super dry (cooked, dried pieces will keep for that long as well). Store the ground chaga in a glass jar in a dry, temperature-controlled spot.*

The boiling time will vary greatly, depending on the strength of the tea desired. If you want a basic, daily drinking brew, 1 hour is enough. If you're looking for a more potent medicinal brew, boil for up to 24 hours. Note that the water will evaporate over time, so if you're brewing for an extended period, continually add water to maintain the liquid level. (Be careful about leaving the boiling chaga unattended because if all the water were to evaporate, the chaga could catch fire.) Turn it off at night; simply cover the pot and resume boiling, uncovered, in the morning. A slow cooker also works if chaperoning your chaga sounds like too much of a commitment.

RECIPES TO REGULATE BLOOD SUGAR

· ·

If you're looking to regulate and stabilize your blood sugar levels, maitake is the best-equipped mushroom for the job. It's not the only one that will work—shiitake, oyster, and reishi are also effective—but it's our go-to for sure. You can easily add or substitute maitake in the recipes we've included in this section that do not directly call for it.

Also, these recipes include carbs. Such a notion might really muddy up the waters as far as what you may be thinking a healthy diet should include. Those carbohydrate-free diets that were all the rage in recent years instilled some seriously carb-phobic ideas, but rest assured that carbohydrates are actually *good* for you. You just need to be carb-smart, meaning you need to select the ones that won't spike your blood sugar the way that so many simple, processed carbohydrates—like white bread, white rice, and all-purpose flour, for example—will. Unprocessed carbohydrates like wild rice ensure optimal nutrients for lasting energy, without any crazy crashes.

Oyster Mushroom Wild Rice Salad

Paleo • Vegan • Gluten-free • Low-glycemic • Low-fat

For this recipe (and any other that calls for wild rice), be sure to buy the best quality rice that you can find and afford. There are countless food marketing scams crammed onto grocery shelves all over the country, so make sure that what you are buying is truly wild rice. In fact, wild rice is actually not "rice" at all, but is derived from four different species of grass, making it infinitely more nutrient-dense than traditional white rice. Wild rice packs immense benefits, from helping with digestion to boosting the immune system, and is also naturally gluten-free and low in calories.

You can easily serve this salad as a satisfying vegetarian main course, but it also makes a nice side dish when served with roasted whole fish or grilled chicken and a simple green salad. It's best when served straight away, but it can also be prepared a day in advance and enjoyed as a chilled lunchtime salad—perfect for a picnic.

SERVES 4 TO 6

TOTAL TIME: 30 TO 50 MINUTES

> 1 tablespoon coconut oil, ghee (see sidebar), or other fat of choice
>
> 2 cups sliced oyster mushrooms
>
> 2 cups wild rice (see Note)
>
> 1/2 cup chopped fresh herbs, such as thyme, oregano, basil, parsley, etc.
>
> 1/2 cup chopped red grapes (can substitute apples, plums, or peaches)
>
> Juice of 1 lemon
>
> 1/4 cup olive oil
>
> 1 cup pecans or walnuts, chopped
>
> Sea salt and freshly ground pepper

1. In a deep stockpot or Dutch oven, melt the coconut oil over medium-high heat. Heat for a minute, then add the mushrooms. Cook, stirring, for 5 to 10 minutes, until the mushrooms are golden brown. Transfer to a plate and set aside.

2. Add the rice and 4 cups water to the pot and raise the heat to high. Bring the water to a boil, then cover and reduce the heat to maintain a simmer. Cook for 40 minutes.

3. Spread the cooked rice over a baking sheet with a spatula and allow it to cool completely.

4. Once the rice has cooled, transfer it to a large bowl and add the mushrooms, herbs, grapes, lemon juice, olive oil, and nuts. Taste and season with salt and pepper. Toss until thoroughly combined and serve immediately. Leftovers can be kept in an airtight container in the refrigerator.

Note • *You can soak the wild rice in 4 cups water for 8 to 12 hours to shorten the cooking time. If you've presoaked the rice, you can use the soaking water as the cooking liquid and reduce the cooking time to 15 minutes.*

What's the Deal with Ghee?

Long a staple in Indian cuisine, ghee (or clarified butter) is made by heating butter for a long time over low heat to separate the butterfat from the milk solids, which are then strained out. The long cooking time produces a nuttier, more robust flavor than in regular butter, and by removing the milk solids, it becomes safe for those with dairy allergies or sensitivities. Other advantages to ghee are its super-long shelf life and the fact that it has a much higher smoke point than

(continued)

butter, which is why we suggest ghee (or oil) in recipes calling for high heat. The main reason we recommend it, however, is that it is richer in vitamins A, D, and E and has a higher percentage of short-chain fatty acids. These fatty acids, in the form of butyric acid, have been shown to stabilize blood sugar, aid with digestion, and decrease inflammation. We're not against using regular butter or cooking oils, and we often give you the option to use what you like and what you have on hand, but if you have time to make your own ghee, it's worth making the switch. If you don't want to make your own ghee, you can find it in the Indian section of many grocery stores or next to the other butter products at natural foods stores.

Raw Vegan Sushi with Shiitake

Paleo • Vegan • Gluten-free • Low-glycemic • Low-fat

This dish is a fresh and fun interpretation of a sushi maki roll and will have all your guests thinking, "You made *sushi*! That must have taken you all day!" In fact, this recipe takes only about 20 minutes to make, so it's minimal effort with a huge payoff.

While most sushi is relatively healthy, it's traditionally made with white rice, which is such a refined starch that it is basically bereft of nutrients. Brown rice is only slightly better on the nutrition scale, so we've devised our own form of sushi rice using crumbled cauliflower. This seasoned, sweet, salty, nutty addition will make you wonder why you ever needed rice in your sushi in the first place! Using vegetables with high fiber and high water content like cauliflower, cucumber, and red pepper in this recipe only adds to the dish's overall effectiveness in stabilizing blood sugar.

SERVES 4

TOTAL TIME: 20 MINUTES

Juice of 1 lemon

2 tablespoons extra-virgin olive oil

1 tablespoon tamari, plus more for serving

½ teaspoon cayenne pepper

10 shiitake mushrooms, stemmed and thinly sliced

1 small head cauliflower, cut into florets

¼ cup pine nuts, lightly toasted

1 tablespoon apple cider vinegar

1 teaspoon sea salt

1 tablespoon pure maple syrup

5 nori sheets (see Note)

½ medium cucumber, peeled and thinly sliced

½ red bell pepper, thinly sliced

Handful of sprouts

Prepared wasabi, for serving

1. In a medium bowl, whisk together the lemon juice, olive oil, tamari, and cayenne. Add the mushrooms to the bowl and set aside.
2. Put the cauliflower florets in a food processor and pulse a few times to break it up, until the cauliflower is evenly crumbly but not mushy.
3. Add the pine nuts, vinegar, salt, and maple syrup to the food processor. Pulse a few times to combine. This is the "rice."
4. Place a nori sheet, shiny-side down, on a dry cutting board or sushi-rolling bamboo mat. Cover the half of the sheet closest to you with a ¼-inch-thick layer of the cauliflower rice. Place a few shiitakes (reserve the marinade), cucumber slices, and pepper slices in a line over the cauliflower layer. Top the vegetables with a handful of sprouts. Roll the sheet gently but firmly, creating a tight log. Repeat with remaining nori and filling.
5. Slice each roll into six even slices. Serve immediately with the reserved tamari marinade and prepared wasabi for dipping.

Note • *Nori are paperlike sheets of pressed seaweed that are available in the Asian section of many grocery stores, specialty food shops, and any Asian market.*

Shiitake Carpaccio

Paleo • Vegetarian • Gluten-free • Low-glycemic • Low-fat

This shiitake carpaccio could win recipe awards across the board: it's insanely easy to prepare, has minimal calories, is packed with nutrients, and is surprisingly satisfying given its simplicity. It's such a well-balanced gastronomic experience and hits all the right notes—there's peppery arugula, brightness from the lemon, hot-and-smoky paprika, and the creamy, salty, umami flavor from the cheese. It's heaven in your mouth, and it's beautiful to boot.

SERVES 2

TOTAL TIME: 10 MINUTES

1 bunch arugula

8 ounces shiitake mushrooms, stemmed and thinly sliced (see Note)

Juice of 1/2 lemon

Extra-virgin olive oil

Salt and freshly ground black pepper

Smoked paprika

1 1/2 ounces shredded Parmesan cheese

Divide the arugula between two plates and top with the mushroom slices. Drizzle the lemon juice and olive oil over the mushrooms. Season with salt, pepper, and paprika and finish with a sprinkling of Parmesan.

Note • *Don't throw out the stems! They are a flavorful addition to vegetable stock.*

Maitake Muffins

Paleo • Gluten-free • Low-fat

We've all accepted that muffins are really just unfrosted cakes disguised as healthy breakfast options when really, they're anything but. These maitake muffins are a much healthier choice. Here, we replaced nutritionally void all-purpose flour with coconut flour and substituted dairy milk with nut milk to cut down on excess sugar (even though the naturally occurring lactose in milk is better for you than table sugar, it can still elevate your blood sugar levels). Swapping in these ingredients allows for the carbohydrates to be released more slowly, so you won't have to worry about a post-sugar crash messing up your morning. These savory muffins are satisfying and intensely flavorful, and are actually good for you, too.

MAKES 18 MUFFINS

TOTAL TIME: 35 MINUTES

1 tablespoon butter, coconut oil, or ghee, plus more for greasing

12 ounces maitake mushrooms, coarsely chopped

1 cup diced onion

1 cup coconut flour

¼ cup cornstarch

1 teaspoon baking powder

1 teaspoon sea salt

½ teaspoon freshly ground black pepper

4 large eggs

3 tablespoons honey

¼ cup almond milk

¼ cup fresh cilantro, chopped

1. Preheat the oven to 400°F. Lightly grease three 6-cup muffin tins.

2. In a skillet, melt the butter over medium heat. Add the mushrooms and onion and cook, stirring frequently, for about 10 minutes, until the mushrooms are golden brown and the onions are slightly caramelized. Set aside to cool.

3. In a large bowl, whisk together the coconut flour, cornstarch, baking powder, salt, and pepper. In a separate bowl, whisk together the eggs, honey, almond milk, and cilantro. Pour the egg mixture into the flour mix and stir well to combine.

4. Add the mushroom and onion mixture to the batter and stir until just combined. Fill the greased muffin pans about three-quarters full. Bake for about 20 minutes, or until a toothpick inserted into the center of a muffin comes out clean. Allow the muffins to cool in the pans for 5 to 10 minutes, then remove and transfer to a wire rack to cool completely.

RECIPES FOR CHRONIC INFLAMMATION

Whether you have an autoimmune disease, a long history of eating white sugar and processed foods, or just have not maintained optimal gut health, chances are that you suffer from some degree of chronic inflammation. You'll know this to be true if you regularly feel gassy or bloated, tired or drained, or just generally not great after many of the meals you eat. Inflammation should be addressed ASAP, before it takes you further down a path that can lead to larger health concerns like obesity, heart disease, or even cancer. But don't worry—the good news is that a proven way to reduce and eliminate chronic inflammation is by making wise and healthful diet decisions. We've got you covered with these dishes that are packed with healing nutrients and stabilizing enzymes.

Chaga Chai

Paleo • Vegan • Gluten-free • Low-glycemic • Low-fat

Chai is positively swimming with health benefits. However, an issue with many commercially available or prepackaged chai blends is that they're polluted with additives and sugars, negating many of chai's healing benefits. But when made from scratch, chai can be extremely good for you. Indian chai is traditionally made with sugar, milk, and/or black tea, but since these ingredients can be hard to digest, we developed a chai recipe using nut milk, for its anti-inflammatory good fats, and coconut palm sugar, which has a much lower glycemic index than white sugar. We've also added ginger for its anti-inflammatory properties, cinnamon and black pepper to increase circulation and boost metabolism, nutmeg to promote good digestion, cardamom to boost your mood, and cloves to activate the potency of the other spices. Adding chaga as the final powerful anti-inflammatory ingredient brings this bevvy to a new, wow-worthy level.

SERVES 6

TOTAL TIME: 15 TO 20 MINUTES

1 (2-inch) piece fresh ginger (or more, if desired), peeled and thinly sliced

10 whole cloves

5 cardamom pods

2 cinnamon sticks

2 teaspoons whole black peppercorns

2 cups nut milk of your choice

1 teaspoon chaga extract

2 tablespoons coconut palm sugar

1. In a medium saucepan, combine the ginger, cloves, cardamom, cinnamon sticks, peppercorns, and 6 cups water. Bring to a boil over

medium heat. Boil for 1 minute, then cover and reduce the heat to low. Simmer for about 10 minutes.

2. Add the nut milk, chaga extract, and coconut palm sugar. Return to a simmer and cook, whisking gently, until the sugar has dissolved. Strain into mugs and serve immediately.

SUGAR, NOT SO SWEET

White sugar has no nutrients, no proteins, no enzymes, and no healthy fats, so it's a gigantic no-no. Since it's one of the most inflammatory things you can consume, regular indulgences can wreak havoc on your digestive system. For one thing, white sugar is considered "free sugar," which means it is not bound to fiber the way that sugar in whole fruits is. Without the fiber to slow digestion, your blood sugar levels get out of whack (which can eventually lead to conditions like diabetes). Here's how: When sugar enters the bloodstream, the pancreas releases insulin to stabilize your blood sugar and the adrenals are triggered to produce extra cortisol. In the digestive system, cortisol inhibits the production of hydrochloric acid, which is required to break down food. This acidic imbalance can lead to chronic inflammation, leaky gut, gas and bloating, and eventually even autoimmune disease. Excess sugar also decreases the body's mineral supply. While coconut palm sugar is not a health food, it does contain many trace minerals and has a lower fructose and glucose content, which means it won't affect your blood sugar as dramatically. Still, use it in moderation and, as always, be sure you are purchasing a quality product.

Maitake Ginger Chews

Paleo • Vegan • Gluten-free • Low-fat

In addition to aiding digestion, ginger helps with inflammation. Ginger contains molecular compounds called gingerols, which are bioactive compounds that reduce the production of excess prostaglandins. Prostaglandins are fats that collect in areas where there is tissue damage or infection, and can cause inflammation and inhibit blood flow, among other things. Maitake has the proven ability to reduce intestinal inflammation, which, when left untreated, can lead to chronic inflammation. Maitake and ginger are a powerful duo when it comes to reducing inflammation and preventing tummy troubles, so toss the Tums and chew on these instead.

MAKES 20 "CHEW BALLS"

TOTAL TIME: 15 MINUTES PLUS 2 HOURS CHILLING TIME

30 small dried dates (about 2 loose cups), soaked in water for 2 hours and drained

1 tablespoon almond butter

3 tablespoons grated fresh ginger (from about one 5-inch piece)

$\frac{1}{2}$ teaspoon pure vanilla extract

$\frac{1}{4}$ teaspoon fine sea salt

3 tablespoons coconut oil

$\frac{1}{2}$ teaspoon liquid stevia

$\frac{1}{2}$ teaspoon ground cinnamon

2 tablespoons maitake extract

$\frac{1}{2}$ cup crushed almonds

1. Using a clean, absorbent kitchen towel, squeeze most of the water out of the soaked dates.
2. Put the dates in a high-speed blender and add the almond butter, ginger, vanilla, salt, coconut oil, stevia, and cinnamon. Blend until

smooth. (A Vitamix or other high-speed blender with a tamper stick works the best for this, but you can also use a food processor fitted with the S-blade.)

3. Form the dough into a large ball and place it in a large bowl. Cover the dough directly with plastic wrap and freeze for 1 hour.

4. Remove the chilled dough from the freezer. Using your hands, pull off bits of dough and roll them into 1-inch balls.

5. In a bowl, combine the maitake extract and the crushed almonds, then spread the mixture on a plate. Roll the chew balls in the coating and transfer to a clean plate. Refrigerate for at least 1 hour before serving. Store the balls in an airtight container in the refrigerator for up to 10 days.

Pickled and Dehydrated Shiitake Jerky

Paleo • Vegan • Gluten-free • Low-glycemic • Low-fat

Pickling is a form of fermentation, a process that naturally infuses the item being pickled with probiotics that generate good bacteria in your gut. While the gut-health-promoting properties and high fiber of these pickles make them great for reducing inflammation, the real bonus about this recipe is that it's a twofer: you can enjoy these mushrooms in their pickled form—they are super good in salads or as a flavorful addition to grain bowls—or you can dehydrate them to make vegetarian jerky for snacking.

MAKES 1 QUART

TOTAL TIME: 40 MINUTES ACTIVE TIME, PLUS PICKLING TIME (3 TO 14 DAYS) AND/OR DEHYDRATING TIME (2 TO 3 HOURS)

> **2 cups dried shiitake mushrooms, or 8 ounces fresh shiitakes, stemmed and thickly sliced**
>
> **½ cup coconut palm sugar**
>
> **½ cup soy sauce**
>
> **½ cup white wine vinegar**
>
> **1 (3-inch) piece fresh ginger, peeled and finely chopped**

1. If using dried mushrooms, soak them in 2 cups hot water for about 20 minutes, or until soft. Remove the mushrooms from the water and squeeze out the extra liquid. Stem the mushrooms and slice the caps into thick strips. Strain the soaking liquid through a fine-mesh sieve lined with a coffee filter set over a saucepan.

2. Add the sugar, soy sauce, vinegar, and ginger to the soaking liquid. Bring the mixture to a boil, then reduce the heat to medium-low and simmer for 20 minutes. Remove the saucepan from the heat and allow the mixture to cool.

3. Put the mushrooms in a 1-quart mason jar. Pour in enough of the cooled soy sauce mixture to cover them. Cover the jar and refrigerate for 3 days and up to 2 weeks, depending on the desired flavor. You can stop here and enjoy the mushrooms as you would any pickle. Or . . .

4. To make jerky, preheat the oven to 150°F. Line a baking sheet with parchment paper.

5. Place the pickled shiitake pieces on the prepared baking sheet and dehydrate in the oven for 2 to 3 hours, keeping the oven door slightly open for ventilation (the handle of a wooden spoon propped in the oven door works well).

Chocolate-Avocado Mousse with Turkey Tail

Vegan • Paleo • Gluten-free • Low-glycemic

This dessert is so simple—and it's addictively good. Need proof? The last time I made this dessert, I ate all four portions by myself. Though I don't recommend making a regular habit of this bulk consumption, it was better for me than eating an entire quart of ice cream (and I know none of us has ever done that, right?).

This mousse is dessert health food across the board. Cacao is incredibly rich in magnesium—one of the most crucial-for-good-health minerals there is—and can do everything from reduce stress to improve heart health. The avocado and nut milk contain anti-inflammatory good fats, and while you could use any medicinal mushroom in this recipe, I particularly like making it with turkey tail, which has extremely effective anti-inflammatory properties.

So give yourself a break the next time you have guests coming for dinner, and make this mousse. You can make it a day or two in advance, and if your guests don't show, trust me when I say you won't have any trouble eating it all by yourself.

SERVES 4

TOTAL TIME: 10 MINUTES, PLUS CHILLING TIME

- $1/2$ cup unsweetened cacao powder
- $1/2$ cup nut milk of choice (almond, hemp, coconut, cashew, etc.)
- 2 teaspoons liquid stevia
- 1 teaspoon turkey tail extract
- 1 teaspoon coconut oil, at room temperature
- 1 teaspoon pure vanilla extract

Pinch of sea salt

2 large ripe avocados, pitted and peeled

Dried fruit, nuts, or seeds of choice (optional)

1. In a small bowl, whisk together the cacao powder, nut milk, stevia, turkey tail extract, coconut oil, vanilla, and salt. Set aside.

2. Place the avocados in a blender and puree until smooth. Add the cacao mixture and blend to incorporate. (If you opt to do this by hand, a handheld mixer will work just as well.)

3. Divide the mousse among four dessert bowls or ramekins. Refrigerate for 1 to 3 hours. Just before serving, top each mousse with dried fruit, nuts, or seeds, if desired. The mousse will keep, covered, in the refrigerator for up to 2 days.

CACAO VS. COCOA

We know! The close spelling can make these ingredients confusing, but there's a big difference between the two. Cocoa powder is made from roasting cocoa beans at high heat before grinding them into a powder, while cacao is made by cold-pressing raw cocoa beans. In both processes, the fat is removed, but with cacao the enzymes and fiber content remain stable, aiding in digestion. The cold-press process also lowers the chance for bitter flavors and other inconsistencies to develop, as can happen with cocoa powder.

RECIPES FOR GUT HEALTH

We often hear the advice to "trust your gut," so keeping your trusty sidekick in tip-top shape by feeding it healthy bacteria is a wise idea. All the recipes in this section will replenish the microbes in your gut to create a healthy and flourishing digestive system. These dishes have stood the test of time—miso soup has been consumed in Asian cultures for centuries, and though many believe sauerkraut to be an eighteenth-century German invention, there's evidence that it's been eaten in China for more than two thousand years, about as long as Eastern cultures have been drinking kombucha. Though it's less well-known in the United States, jun tea has a long history of being passed down from generation to generation in Tibetan and Indian cultures. The point is, while we've been busy destroying our guts with refined and processed foods, older civilizations around the world have long understood the importance of eating foods that are restorative to the digestive process. And like we said, good gut health is often the domino that starts the process to overall optimal health.

We've used reishi in two of the four recipes here, but feel free to experiment with other medicinal mushrooms, too, as most, if not all, have incredible gut-healing properties. When it comes to your gut, mushrooms are always a good idea.

Miso Mushroom Seaweed Soup

Paleo • Vegan • Gluten-free • Low-glycemic • Low-fat

Japanese miso soups are known for being low in calories, high in protein, and extremely healthy—studies have even shown that the consumption of miso soup can reduce the incidence of breast cancer. Miso is a paste made out of fermented soybeans. The fermentation process creates good bacteria in the form of probiotics and gives miso its unique umami flavor. If you have a sensitivity to soy products, you can still enjoy this soup; miso can also be made with barley and chickpeas, so shop around to find the option that works for you.

Our twist on miso soup ups the ante on liquid health, thanks to a hearty addition of chaga, seaweed, and almonds. Your bloodstream absorbs nutrients more readily from liquid foods instead of solid foods, so this soup immediately delivers high quantities of probiotics, fiber, protein, and good fats. We're going to guess that the layers of flavor will soon have you serving up seconds, so maybe make a double batch.

SERVES 4

TOTAL TIME: 10 MINUTES PREP TIME PLUS 1 TO 4 HOURS STEEPING TIME (DEPENDING ON PERSONAL PREFERENCE)

2 tablespoons chaga powder

¼ cup unpasteurized miso (soy, barley, or chickpea)

4 garlic cloves

¼ cup extra-virgin olive oil

⅓ cup whole almonds (preferably soaked for at least 4 hours)

¼ cup seaweed flakes (available at natural food and other specialty stores)

Juice of 1 lime

Pinch of chile powder or dash of Sriracha sauce (optional)

Slivered almonds, for garnish (optional)

1. In a large saucepan, combine the chaga powder and 8 cups water. Bring to a simmer over low heat. Simmer for 1 to 4 hours, depending on how strong you want the chaga flavor (see Tip). Keep an eye on the broth as it simmers and add more water as it evaporates.

2. Once the chaga brew reaches your desired potency level, allow it to cool slightly before pouring it into a high-speed blender. Add the miso, garlic, olive oil, whole almonds, seaweed, lime juice, and chili powder and blend on high speed until the soup is smooth and frothy. Be super careful when blending hot liquids—blend the soup in batches, if necessary.

3. Divide the soup among four soup bowls or large mugs and garnish with sliced almonds and additional chili, if desired.

Tip: The stronger the chaga flavor (the longer the chaga steeps in the hot water), the more nutrients the soup will contain.

Mushroom Sauerkraut

Paleo • Vegan • Gluten-free • Low-glycemic • Low-fat

Sauerkraut is a powerhouse of good-for-you bacteria and fiber. It's basically a condiment cure-all for your gut. A few things you need to know about sauerkraut: One, it is one of the most absurdly easy and super-cheap superfoods you can make. Two, it keeps in the fridge for ages. Really, everyone should have a big ol' jar of it constantly chilling out next to the hot sauces, mustards, and pickles currently crowding all refrigerator doors. Three, it's a fun DIY project to make with your kids or friends.

Sauerkraut has long been a staple in Slavic countries, Germany, and Scandinavia. These are also some of the world's most mushroom-friendly countries, and since mushrooms and kraut both offer amazing immune support, eating them together makes sense. You won't necessarily taste the mushrooms in this dish—thanks to sauerkraut's signature sour flavor, you can easily "hide" fairly large quantities of mushrooms, giving you a green light to load up on the reishi, shiitake, or other mushroom of your choice.

MAKES 1 GALLON (ABOUT 25 SERVINGS)

**TOTAL TIME: 30 TO 40 MINUTES PLUS FERMENTATION TIME
(A MINIMUM OF 1 TO 16 WEEKS AND UP TO 1 YEAR)**

SPECIAL EQUIPMENT: Water-sealed fermentation crock/fermenter (strongly recommended) or multiple large mason jars (see Note)

5 pounds thinly sliced cabbage (2 or 3 heads), rinsed and dried

2 red onions, thinly sliced

3 tablespoons salt

2 to 3 teaspoons preferred mushroom extract (reishi and shiitake are especially recommended)

Cayenne pepper, ground turmeric, ground ginger, ground coriander or mustard seeds, as desired (optional)

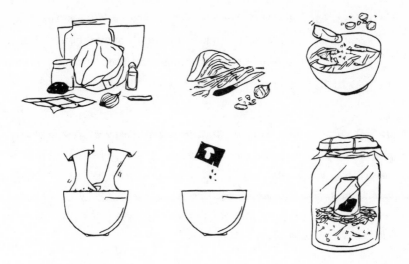

1. Combine the cabbage, onion, and salt in a very large bowl. Massage the mixture with your hands for a few minutes, until the vegetables become limp and release their liquid. The mixture should reduce by about half.

2. Add the mushroom extract and other spices, if using.

3. If you're using a fermentation crock, follow the manufacturer's instructions, making sure the cabbage is completely submerged underneath the weighted plates. If you're using a sterilized mason jar, you can make your own weight by using a smaller sterilized jelly jar filled with pie weights, small stones, or something else to give it heft (see illustration). Once the jelly jar is weighing down the cabbage, cover the larger mason jar with a clean cloth and secure it with a rubber band. Do not use the lid, as it will prevent airflow.

4. The length of fermentation will be anywhere from 1 to 16 weeks, depending on the room temperature, size of your batch (smaller batches and those made in mason jars will ferment much more quickly), and desired flavor. The amount of good bacteria present

will vary and increase over time, but you can safely test the sauerkraut after 1 week and continue to do so daily or weekly, until it is to your liking. Once you obtain your desired flavor, cover the mason jar with its lid and store in the refrigerator for up to 1 year.

Note • If you opt to use a mason jar, be aware that smaller pieces of cabbage can more easily escape the makeshift weight and float up to the top of the liquid. This can create mold. One way to solve this problem is to set aside a few larger outer cabbage leaves and use them to cover the sliced cabbage. The weight goes on top of the outer leaves, which will help keep the cabbage underneath submerged. The outer leaves should be discarded when the sauerkraut is ready to eat.

Reishi Kombucha

Paleo • Vegan • Gluten-free • Low-fat

In Russian, Chinese, and Japanese, *kombucha* literally translates to "tea mushroom," because of the sea creature–esque "mushroom" that floats along the bottom of this tea-based drink. The floater isn't a mushroom but a SCOBY (symbiotic culture of bacteria and yeast), and is the home for the bacteria and yeast that transform tea into kombucha. Every new batch of kombucha creates a "baby" SCOBY, so the best way to get started making

ing kombucha on your own is to receive an extra SCOBY from a friend. You can also start a batch from an unpasteurized, store-bought kombucha drink—just set aside the tiny SCOBY and ½ to 1 cup of the kombucha before drinking it and store together in a tightly sealed bag or jar filled with sugar water in the fridge.

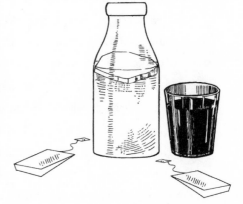

Because kombucha is fermented, it will have a very slight alcohol content. If prepared and stored as we indicate here, it will be 0.5% or less.

Feeding a SCOBY

A quick note about the sugar in this recipe, since we know white sugar is the enemy: The SCOBY feeds on sugar, and it's necessary to create the essential probiotics that make kombucha so valuable for promoting gut health. The fermentation process will break down the sugar, so the longer the kombucha ferments, the less sugar will be in the final product—just a fraction of the sugar you began with.

MAKES 8 CUPS

TOTAL TIME: 20 MINUTES PLUS FERMENTATION TIME (7 TO 10 DAYS)

4 bags of black tea

2 grams reishi extract powder

1/2 cup sugar

1 cup minimally flavored prepared kombucha drink (can be store-bought)

1 kombucha SCOBY (from the prepared drink)

1. Bring 1 cup water to a boil in a large saucepan. Add the tea bags, turn off the heat, and steep for 5 minutes.

2. Remove and discard the tea bags. Stir in the reishi extract powder and sugar.

3. Add 7 cups water to the sweetened reishi-tea mixture to cool it down. Transfer the liquid to a large sterilized mason jar.

4. Add the prepared kombucha drink as a starter, then gently place the SCOBY on top (the starter tea should always be at least 10 percent of the drink you're making, since without the SCOBY and starter, your kombucha will not have the bacterial base to grow from). The SCOBY may float or sink—after a few days, it should start floating or a new SCOBY will begin to form on top of the liquid.

5. Cover the mouth of the jar with a clean cloth and secure it in place with an elastic band. Let the jar stand at room temperature, out of direct sunlight, for 7 to 10 days. Taste the kombucha every few days to see how the flavor changes. When you like the flavor, remove the SCOBY and save it in an airtight container filled with sugar water in the fridge for your next batch. Decant the kombucha in small glass bottles (see Note).

Note • *If you prefer your kombucha carbonated, add an additional teaspoon of sugar to each bottle, seal them tightly, and let stand at room temperature for an additional 2 days before transferring them to the fridge.*

 ADVANCED MOVE

Try making kombucha from oolong or Pu-erh teas. Oolong is a happy medium between black tea and green tea, while Pu-erh, on the other hand, is a very strong fermented tea from China's Yunnan province. We recommend trying oolong first, as Pu-erh has a deep, earthy flavor that is something of an acquired taste. It's worth experimenting with both as they contain significant health benefits that go beyond those of typical black breakfast tea.

Mushroom Jun Tea

Paleo • Vegetarian • Gluten-free • Low-fat

Jun tea is kombucha's lesser-known Tibetan cousin. Unlike its more popular relative, jun tea feeds on honey instead of sugar and has a green tea
base. Both offer similar gut-healing probiotic benefits, but jun tea's flavor
is a bit smoother, so it can be a more appealing option for those who are
just starting out with fermented teas. Kombucha is fantastic, but because
honey is preferable to sugar in terms of health and green tea is packed with
such an array of antioxidants, it's only a matter of time before jun tea takes
over the health beverage spotlight.

Jun tea usually contains a higher alcohol content (around 2%, compared to
kombucha's possible 0.5%), so you might not want to serve it to children.
This recipe calls for lion's mane extract, but you can also experiment with
other mushroom extracts.

MAKES 1 GALLON (8 TO 10 SERVINGS)

TOTAL TIME: 10 MINUTES PLUS FERMENTATION TIME (3 TO 10 DAYS)

6 to 8 teaspoons loose-leaf green tea of your choice

1 cup raw honey

1 jun culture (SCOBY; see sidebar on page 108)

2 teaspoons lion's mane extract

Starter jun tea

1. Bring 1 gallon spring water to a boil in a large pot and add the green
   tea. Remove from the heat and allow the tea to steep for 5 to 10 minutes. Let cool to lukewarm.
2. Add the honey to the lukewarm tea and steep for 10 minutes more.
3. Strain the tea to remove the leaves and allow it to cool to room
   temperature.

4. Transfer the tea to a large sterile mason jar and add the jun SCOBY, lion's mane extract, and the starter tea (this should always be about 10 percent by volume of the drink you're making, as without the SCOBY and starter tea, your jun will not have the bacterial base needed for fermentation).

5. Cover the mouth of the jar with a clean cloth and secure it in place with an elastic band. Store the jun tea at room temperature out of direct sunlight. Depending on your environment, your SCOBY, and the storage jar used, jun tea can take anywhere from 3 to 10 days to ferment. There's no precise science on the amount of time, so test it along the way. Take your first sample after 3 days, and keep trying once each day until it tastes right to you. The tangier it tastes, the stronger it is, and the less sugar remains from the honey.

6. When you're happy with the flavor, remove and store the SCOBY in sugar water in the fridge. Decant the tea into smaller glass bottles. Once bottled, the tea can sit for an additional 2 to 3 days at room temperature to create some slight carbonation. You can also transfer the bottles directly to the refrigerator, which will immediately stop the fermentation process. Bottled mushroom jun tea will keep in the refrigerator for up to 1 month.

 ADVANCED MOVE

Try making Mushroom Jun Tea with half green tea and half yerba mate or gua-yusa. The end result is a highly caffeinated beverage that will give you a serious fermented energy boost.

Fermented Beginnings

If you don't have a SCOBY from a past batch or a fellow fermenter, you can use store-bought bottled kombucha or jun tea. Once you start making your own, always remember to save some of the drink to use as a starter for your next batch. After a few batches, you will actually grow a new SCOBY, which you can donate to a friend. You can cut bigger SCOBYs into smaller pieces to run several batches at the same time, but minimize the handling of the SCOBY with your bare hands and don't use metallic instruments to cut it (a ceramic knife is the best option).

RECIPES FOR HORMONAL BALANCE

· ·

The human body produces more than fifty hormones, so it's not surprising that the balance often gets tipped in one direction or another. Normal hormonal activity can be disrupted by environmental, physical, or emotional changes; aging; an increase in stress levels; and as a result of the various uppers and downers many of us consistently ingest in the form of food and drink, vitamins and supplements, and prescribed medications. Due to the culture we live in, it's not too surprising that the vast majority of hormonal imbalances most people suffer from are related to being *over*stimulated. This point can easily be driven home when you consider how many times people mention how stressed, busy, or tired they are during an average week.

We're not saying your morning mug of coffee or your evening glass of red is a no-no, but we do suggest that you try mushroom coffee and mushroom cocktails as alternatives (see pages 153–59 and 173–78). The real issue is that you should not be relying on using uppers throughout the day to the point where you have to counteract their effects with a slew of downers at night to mellow out. Your body doesn't deserve such a constant roller coaster ride! In fact, your body won't allow it and will rebel in all kinds of nasty ways (in the form of weight gain, loss of sex drive, poor digestion, that awful wired/tired yo-yo dance, and more). Fortunately, the recipes we include here will keep all your hormones balanced and in check.

Turkey-Tail Carob Elixir

Paleo • Vegan • Gluten-free • Low-glycemic • Low-fat

The comfort that comes from enjoying a warm, delicious beverage is something everyone should be able to experience, but some people's systems are too sensitive to handle the stimulants that are naturally present in coffee, hot chocolate, and most teas. This recipe takes care of that problem. We use carob powder, which contains none of the caffeine or theobromine found in coffee and cacao, so there will be absolutely no jitters or diuretic effects to worry about. While you won't fully confuse the flavor of carob for that of chocolate or coffee, you'll still taste the essence of both, so it makes for a satisfying alternative. The big bonus here is that without having to deal with any stimulation to the nervous system, the body can better absorb the nutrients from the carob and turkey tail mushroom. We added turkey tail for its adaptogenic properties, making this elixir a great choice for anyone with adrenal fatigue or overall elevated stress levels. Try it first without the maple syrup; you may find this hearty, earthy, energizing beverage is just right as it is.

SERVES 4

TOTAL TIME: 5 MINUTES

¼ cup carob powder

¼ cup unsweetened desiccated coconut

¼ cup almonds (preferably soaked in water for at least 4 hours)

2 teaspoons coconut oil

1 teaspoon turkey tail extract (see Note)

1 teaspoon ground cinnamon

½ vanilla bean, seeds scraped and pod discarded

2 to 3 tablespoons pure maple syrup, agave, raw honey, or other natural sweetener (optional)

Combine all the ingredients and 3 cups hot water in a high-speed blender and blend on high until completely combined and smooth, 15 to 20 seconds. Divide among four mugs and serve immediately.

Note • *Instead of using the turkey tail extract, you can make your own turkey tail decoction by soaking 3 to 5 pieces in 5 to 6 cups hot water for 4 to 5 hours.*

Reishi Chocolate Almonds

Paleo • Vegetarian • Gluten-free

Thanks to the healthy fats in the almonds, the natural sweetness of the honey, and the metabolism-boosting properties of cinnamon, these are chocolate-covered nuts you can feel good about eating. When shopping for dark chocolate, choose the brand with the highest cacao percentage you can find and afford, as it will contain fewer sugars, milk solids, and additives. And as for the reishi, it's the best mushroom to reach for at night—its adaptogenic properties work to calm your system and ensure quality, restful sleep, so it's a great snack to have before bedtime.

SERVES 4 TO 6

TOTAL TIME: 20 MINUTES

6 ounces dark chocolate (at least 70 to 80% cacao)

1 teaspoon reishi mushroom extract powder

⅓ cup raw honey

Pinch of ground cinnamon

1 cup raw almonds (unblanched; preferably soaked for at least 4 hours)

1. Line a baking sheet with parchment paper.
2. Melt the chocolate in a double boiler over low heat, about 10 minutes. Add the reishi powder to the melted chocolate, stir well to combine, and set aside.
3. Meanwhile, in a saucepan, combine the honey, cinnamon, and ⅓ cup water. Bring to a simmer over medium heat. When the mixture begins to simmer, stir in the almonds. Cook the nuts for 5 minutes, stirring occasionally. Remove from the heat.

4. Add the honey-coated almonds to the chocolate and stir until evenly coated. Spread the chocolate-covered almonds over the prepared baking sheet and set aside to cool, allowing them to harden for at least 1 hour before serving.

Superfood Slushie

Paleo • Vegan • Gluten-free

This spoonable meal is packed with antioxidants, delivering energy and nutrients to your body to keep you going for hours. Made with healing herbs, it has powerful adaptogenic properties, and—best of all—can be changed up daily to suit your tastes and preferences. I've been making some variation on this slushie almost every day for breakfast or as an afternoon snack for the past ten years. Consider it an edible playground and an opportunity to have some fun in the kitchen. But make sure to rinse well with water or give your teeth a good brushing afterward—a big green smile is not a good look on anyone!

MAKES 1 BOWL

TOTAL TIME: 3 MINUTES

1 tablespoon spirulina powder

2 tablespoons honey

2 tablespoons olive oil

1 tablespoon hulled hemp seeds

1 teaspoon reishi or chaga extract

Pinch of salt

Preferred toppings (dried inca, goji berries, blueberries, cacao nibs, bee pollen, sliced avocado, nuts, and/or seeds)

Mix all the ingredients except the toppings with ½ cup water in a bowl. Finish with a sprinkling of the toppings of your choice.

Maca-Mushroom Buns

Vegan • Gluten-free • Low-fat

Maca is a wonder drug when it comes to restoring and regulating the hormonal system. It's celebrated for helping women regain their libido, which is why it's best known for its powers as an aphrodisiac. Adding maitake for its blood-regulating properties means you won't need to worry about a carb crash. These buns have a chewy texture that's as satisfying and delicious as traditional rolls, and they can easily be made gluten-free depending on the oats you use.

MAKES 12 BUNS

TOTAL TIME: 1 HOUR

> 1 cup old-fashioned rolled oats (use certified gluten-free oats if necessary for your diet)
>
> 11 grams instant yeast (about 2 heaping teaspoons, depending on the brand)
>
> 2 cups lukewarm water
>
> 2 cups gluten-free all-purpose flour
>
> 6 tablespoons maca root powder
>
> 2 tablespoons maitake mushroom powder
>
> 1 teaspoon salt
>
> 1 tablespoon coconut sugar
>
> 3 tablespoons olive oil
>
> Flaxseeds, as desired (optional)

1. Preheat the oven to 450°F and position a rack in the center of the oven. Line a baking sheet with parchment paper.
2. In a large bowl, stir together the oats, yeast, and 2 cups lukewarm water.

3. Add the flour, maca, maitake, salt, coconut sugar, and olive oil and stir with a wooden spoon until evenly mixed. Pour onto the prepared baking sheet and shape into a rectangle. Cover with a clean kitchen towel and let rise for 30 minutes.

4. Sprinkle the dough with a bit of water and scatter flaxseeds on top, if desired. Use a knife to slice the dough into 12 equal squares, but keep the squares together. Bake for 12 to 15 minutes, or until golden brown. Transfer to a wire rack and let cool slightly before serving.

RECIPES FOR IMMUNE SUPPORT

· ·

The heart of this book lies in mushrooms' ability to offer incredible immune support. No matter which mushroom(s) you choose to add to your life, your immune system will benefit greatly, and an optimally functioning immune system will lead to great overall health and wellness. All the mushrooms we discuss in this book contain crucial polysaccharides and beta-glucans that make them powerful immunomodulators, though each works slightly differently in the body. Basically, cooking with mushrooms will help you feel your best. Here we've chosen some of our all-time favorite recipes for that very reason.

Broccoli Soup with Mushroom "Bacon"

Paleo • Vegan • Gluten-free

Pairing a superfood like shiitake with broccoli—which has been called "the world's healthiest vegetable" due to its ample amounts of fiber, vitamins, and nutrients—makes this soup something of a wonder bowl. In addition to delivering a dose of shiitake's beauty benefits (glowing skin!), this soup is incredibly creamy (despite being completely dairy-free), has a great crunch from the vegan "bacon," and gets a nice kick from the raw onion. This is a vegan and vegetarian crowd-pleaser for sure, but we bet it'll be the carnivores at the table serving themselves up seconds. Adding the shiitake extract is not mandatory, but is highly recommended to make the soup more potent.

SERVES 6

TOTAL TIME: 45 MINUTES

FOR THE MUSHROOM BACON
¼ cup sunflower oil

1 smoked sweet paprika

2 teaspoons coarsely ground cumin

3 tablespoons pure maple syrup

1 teaspoon shiitake powder (optional)

Salt and freshly ground black pepper

12 shiitake mushrooms

FOR THE BROCCOLI SOUP
2 large heads broccoli, chopped into florets

3 carrots, coarsely chopped

3 celery stalks, coarsely chopped

1 medium onion, coarsely chopped

1 cup cashews (preferably soaked in water for at least 4 hours)

3 tablespoons coconut butter or ghee

3 tablespoons olive oil

2 teaspoons salt

1 teaspoon freshly ground black pepper

1. To make the bacon, preheat the oven to 350°F. Line a baking sheet with aluminum foil.

2. In a medium bowl, stir together the sunflower oil, paprika, cumin, syrup, and shiitake powder (if using) until combined. Season with salt and pepper.

3. Stem the mushrooms, reserving the stems for the soup. Slice the caps into ½-inch-thick slices and place them flat on the prepared baking sheet. Drizzle with three-quarters of the syrup mixture and toss to coat. Bake for 15 to 20 minutes, until golden brown.

4. Remove the baking sheet from the oven, flip the mushrooms, and pour the remaining syrup mixture on top. Bake for 10 to 15 minutes more, or until the mushrooms are crispy. Remove from the oven and set aside to cool.

5. Meanwhile, to make the soup, bring 4 cups water to a boil in a large pot. Add the broccoli, carrots, celery, and reserved mushroom stems and cook until soft, 5 to 7 minutes.

6. Add the onion, cashews, coconut butter, olive oil, salt, and pepper. Carefully puree the soup directly in the pot with an immersion blender until smooth.

7. Divide the soup among six bowls and top with the mushroom bacon.

Chaga Jelly Bowl

Paleo • Gluten-free • Low-fat

I know this recipe sounds weird: Who wants to eat a bowl of jelly? Well, once you hear what's in this bowl of goodness—which has the consistency of a thick yogurt and makes for a great breakfast, snack, or dessert—you sure will. Gelatin is a protein derived from the collagen found in animal bones (so take note that this dish is not vegetarian, but you can make it so by using agar agar instead, and while we have plenty of collagen in our bodies, it's a protein that reduces over time, leading to brittle hair, loss of skin elasticity, and joint problems. The gelatin in this dish can assist with everything from strengthening your hair and nails to providing relief from arthritis. The addition of chaga, which you now know contains ample amounts of melanin to make your skin, hair, and nails positively lustrous, means this jelly bowl might as well be called a beauty bowl. Its beautifying properties aside, this is a simple, easy-to-digest meal that can be customized to satisfy sweet or savory cravings. The immunomodulating benefits are immediate and powerful; you will feel good after eating this.

SERVES 2 GENEROUSLY
TOTAL TIME: 10 MINUTES PLUS 2 HOURS SETTING TIME

1 tablespoon gelatin powder

¼ cup boiled water

1½ cups strong Chaga Decoction (page 74; see Note), cooled

¼ cup honey

OPTIONAL TOPPINGS
Chopped nuts

Seeds

Pine pollen

Gluten-free granola

Fresh berries

Lemon zest

1. In a large bowl, bloom the gelatin by sprinkling it over ½ cup luke-warm water. Let stand for 3 to 5 minutes.
2. Pour the boiling water over the gelatin and whisk well to ensure the gelatin is completely dissolved.
3. Add the chaga decoction and honey and stir to combine. Divide the mixture between two bowls and refrigerate for at least 2 hours to set.
4. When ready to serve, top each bowl with a mix of your preferred toppings.

Note • *If you do not have a batch of Chaga Decoction on hand, you can dissolve 2 grams chaga extract powder in ½ cup hot water. Once fully dissolved, add 1 cup cold water and stir to combine.*

Oyster Mushroom Risotto

Vegetarian • Low-fat

I've eaten my way around the world, and while I've found that the cuisine of every culture is rife with delicacies, it's just hard to top Italian food. There's something about it that is universally appealing; it's always super fresh, rich, and flavorful, yet never too heavy. Italians just get food.

You can bring a taste of *la dolce vita* into your own kitchen with this surprisingly simple risotto recipe. The health bonus here is that oyster mushrooms contain high amounts of ergothioneine, an amino acid and powerful antioxidant that works to protect cells from damage by free radicals and boosts and regulates the body's immune response. This is a health-infused comfort food dish that works well for lunch or dinner, as a main or a side. People can't get enough of it—must be an Italian thing.

SERVES 4

TOTAL TIME: 40 MINUTES

4 cups vegetable, chicken, or beef stock

1 ounce dried oyster mushrooms, or 3 large fresh oyster mushrooms, sliced

2 tablespoons extra-virgin olive oil

2 garlic cloves, finely chopped

1 medium onion, chopped

10 ounces Arborio rice

½ cup dry white wine

4 tablespoons (½ stick) unsalted butter

3 tablespoons grated Parmesan cheese

Small bunch fresh parsley, finely chopped

Salt and freshly ground black pepper

1. In a large pot, bring the stock to a boil over high heat. Turn off the heat, add the dried mushrooms (if using), and cover. Soak for 20 minutes. Remove the mushrooms with a slotted spoon and use a clean kitchen towel to gently squeeze out any excess liquid. Reserve the stock and the mushrooms separately.

2. In a large saucepan, heat the olive oil over medium heat. When the oil is hot, about 1 minute, add the garlic and onion. Cook, stirring continuously, for about 5 minutes, until the garlic and onion are soft and fragrant.

3. Add the rice to the pan and cook for 1 minute. Add the wine and bring to a simmer. Cook for 2 to 3 minutes.

4. Add one-quarter of the reserved stock and simmer, stirring often, until the rice has absorbed all the liquid. Add another quarter of the stock, simmer, and stir until all liquid has been absorbed. Repeat this process with the remaining stock. The total simmering time will be 15 to 20 minutes, and the rice should be just *al dente*.

5. Remove the pan from the heat and stir in the butter, half the cheese, half the parsley, and the rehydrated mushrooms (or the fresh mushrooms, if using), and season with salt and pepper.

6. To serve, spoon the rice onto plates and garnish with the remaining cheese and parsley.

Oatmeal Cookies with Enoki White Chocolate Coating

Vegetarian • Gluten-free

By now, everyone knows about the heart-health benefits of whole oats, so they were a good starting point for this recipe. We added good fats in the form of nuts and nut butter and lowered the glycemic index of the cookies by using coconut palm sugar in place of white sugar. The coating is made with rice bran solubles (tocotrienols), natural sweeteners, and pure cacao butter, making it the healthiest frosting you'll ever eat. Cacao butter contains none of the stimulants found in milk and dark chocolate, so there'll be no caffeine or sugar high with this treat. Adding enoki for its antioxidants like ergothioneine seals the deal on these super cookies. So there's really only one question to ask now: Would you like a glass of warm nut milk with your cookies?

MAKES 30 COOKIES

TOTAL TIME: 30 MINUTES PLUS 20 MINUTES CHILLING TIME

FOR THE COOKIES
½ cup (1 stick) unsalted butter, at room temperature

1 cup almond butter

1 cup coconut palm sugar

2 large eggs

1 teaspoon pure vanilla extract

3 cups old-fashioned rolled oats

1 ½ teaspoons baking soda

½ cup chopped walnuts

FOR THE WHITE CHOCOLATE COATING
1 cup cacao butter

¾ cup tocotrienols (rice bran solubles; see sidebar, page 126)

2 tablespoons lucuma powder (see sidebar, page 126; optional)

2 tablespoons coconut palm sugar

3 grams enoki extract powder

1½ teaspoons pure vanilla extract

Pinch of salt

1. To make the cookies, preheat the oven to 350°F and position the racks in the upper and lower thirds of the oven. Line two baking sheets with parchment paper.

2. In a large bowl using a handheld mixer, beat the butter, almond butter, and coconut palm sugar until smooth.

3. Add the eggs and vanilla and beat until well combined.

4. Using a wooden spoon, mix in the oats and baking soda by hand until just combined. Stir in the walnuts.

5. Drop 2-tablespoon-size portions of dough a few inches apart on the prepared baking sheets.

6. Bake the cookies for 10 to 12 minutes, or until golden brown. Let cool for 5 minutes on the baking sheets before transferring to a wire rack to cool completely.

7. To make the white chocolate coating, chop the cacao butter into large chunks and place in a double boiler over low heat. Melt slowly, until it is completely smooth. Stir in the tocotrienols, lucuma powder (if using), coconut palm sugar, enoki extract powder, vanilla, and salt and mix until well combined. Place the cacao mixture in the refrigerator for 10 minutes to cool slightly.

8. Line a baking sheet with waxed paper. Once the cookies have cooled completely, dip them in the cacao frosting to coat. Place the dipped cookies on the prepared baking sheet and freeze for 20 minutes to set the frosting before serving.

9. Store the remaining cookies in an airtight container at room temperature for up to 4 to 5 days, or in the refrigerator for 2 to 3 weeks.

What Are Tocotrienols?

Tocotrienols are members of the vitamin E family and are found in many fruits and plants like rice, wheat, barley, and rye. We love adding tocotrienol powder to soups, smoothies, desserts, and sauces, as the powder lends a luscious creamy texture without needing to add any dairy products, making this one very healthy secret ingredient. Tocos are an especially helpful supplement for anyone who wants to improve their skin or is sick often.

What Is Lucuma Powder?

This Peruvian fruit can be used in recipes as a natural sweetener. Because it contains vitamins and minerals such as beta-carotene, iron, zinc, vitamin B_3, calcium, and protein, we endorse using it in place of sugar (or at least replacing half the sugar in many recipes with lucuma) for some added essential nutrients. The powdered form can be found at health food stores and online. If you cannot find lucuma powder, simply double the amount of coconut palm sugar.

RECIPES FOR
SKIN AND BEAUTY

· ·

We don't subscribe to specific beauty standards, but it's a basic truth that when everything inside your body is functioning at optimal levels, you will truly be your most beautiful self. Whatever your size, shape, or age, when you have glowing skin, sparkling eyes, and strong, shiny hair and nails, you'll look and feel terrific. We've included these beauty recipes that keep those things in mind.

Chaga Skin Cream

Paleo • Vegan

Funguys can get a little woo-woo sometimes, so we've got a recipe for making your own kick-butt skin cream. It makes sense that the best topical skin care creams often contain the same ingredients you eat for optimal health, since they're directly absorbed into your body. High-quality oils and butters pair perfectly with chaga's incredibly high melanin content and range of antioxidants to create a wonderfully nourishing cream for your skin. This recipe will heal and protect your body's largest organ, leaving you looking and feeling fantastic. You can modify the recipe as desired by adding the essential oils that will best address your particular skin care needs.

MAKES 3 OUNCES
TOTAL TIME: 1 HOUR

1 tablespoon cacao butter

3 tablespoons shea butter

2 tablespoons coconut oil

10 drops essential oils of your choice (see Note)

1 teaspoon chaga extract powder

1. In a double boiler, combine the cacao butter, shea butter, and coconut oil and melt over low heat until smooth. Be careful not to overheat this mixture; you only want to warm it enough to slowly melt everything together.
2. Stir in the essential oil(s). Sprinkle in the chaga extract powder and whisk until well combined. Pour the cream into a glass jar and refrigerate for 30 minutes. Use as desired, especially before and after sun exposure. Store at room temperature. When stored in dry conditions out of direct sunlight, the cream will keep for 1 to 2 years.

Note • *Choose Your Essential Oils:*

Calm down with chamomile and lavender.

Feel positive with patchouli and jasmine.

Get energized with grapefruit and peppermint.

Boost concentration with eucalyptus and rosemary.

Clear your skin with lemon and rose.

Berry Blast Smoothie

Paleo • Vegan • Gluten-free • Low-fat

Berries are so beautifully vibrant in color because they contain ample amounts of flavonoids, a type of polyphenol. When ingested, these compounds serve a number of extraordinary health purposes, including regulating blood sugar and blood pressure levels, inhibiting the spread of cancerous cells, warding off dementia, reducing inflammation, and offering powerful antiaging properties to create glowing, radiant skin. We've added tremella here to take advantage of its impressive hydrating and skin-protecting attributes, but you can play around with other mushrooms, too. This recipe is so easy to whip up that it would be silly not to incorporate it into your daily routine. And when people ask how you came to look so good, you can simply answer that you're just having a blast.

MAKES 4 CUPS, OR 2 LARGE SMOOTHIES
TOTAL TIME: 5 MINUTES

3 cups fresh or frozen berries

1 small pear, cored

3 tablespoons organic nut butter (almond, cashew, hemp, etc.)

3 tablespoons tocotrienols (see sidebar, page 126)

2 tablespoons coconut oil

2 teaspoons tremella extract

Pinch of salt

Combine all the ingredients and 3 cups water in a high-speed blender and blend on high for about 30 seconds, or until completely smooth. Pour into two glasses and serve immediately.

ADVANCED MOVE

Add 1 tablespoon high–vitamin C berry powder (such as camu camu or acerola) to boost collagen production or 1 teaspoon of the superberry schisandra. In China, where schisandra has long been valued for its beautifying properties, shisandra is known as the "quintessence of tonic herbs" for the crazy amounts of antioxidants it contains.

Vegetarian "Clam" Chowder

Paleo • Vegetarian • Gluten-free • Low-glycemic

The name of the game with this recipe is hydration, and this soup offers restorative and regenerative properties by the ladleful. While many soups contain scary amounts of sodium that cause water retention and bloating, this heavenly and hearty number has the opposite effect—you'll feel and look great after chowing down on this chowder. Adding the oyster mushrooms at the end gives them just enough time to acquire a desirable clamlike bite, so even omnivores will enjoy this vegetarian version. We've chosen to use tremella in this recipe because it contains a polysaccharide that can hold up to five hundred times its weight in water (see page 67 for more on that!), and tremella also stimulates the production of the antioxidant superoxide dismutase (SOD), which protects the skin from free radicals. Destination glowing skin, here we come.

SERVES 4

TOTAL TIME: 45 MINUTES

2 cups chopped cauliflower florets

1½ cups almond milk

2 tablespoons unsalted butter

1 yellow onion, thinly sliced

2 celery stalks, cut into medium dice

2 carrots, cut into medium dice

1 tablespoon ground cumin

3 tablespoons cornstarch

2 cups vegetable broth (see Notes)

1 large Yukon Gold or purple potato, peeled and cubed

4 ounces fresh shiitake or oyster mushrooms (see Notes), sliced

1 teaspoon tremella extract

Salt and freshly ground black pepper

1. Fill a stockpot with a steamer basket with 2 inches of water and set over medium-high heat. Place the steamer basket in the pot and bring the water to a boil. Add the cauliflower, cover, and steam for 5 to 7 minutes, or until the cauliflower is tender. Remove the steamer basket and cauliflower, and reserve the cooking water.

2. Transfer the cooked cauliflower to a high-speed blender and add 1 cup of the almond milk and 1 cup of the steaming liquid. Carefully blend until smooth. The mixture will be very hot, so allow some steam to escape while blending, if possible. Set aside.

3. In a stockpot, melt the butter over medium-low heat. Add the onion, celery, carrots, and cumin. Cook, stirring often, until the onions become slightly caramelized, about 15 minutes.

4. Add the cornstarch and stir until completely combined. Add the remaining ¼ cup almond milk, the broth, and the potato. Bring the mixture to a boil. Keep the chowder at a rolling boil for 15 minutes.

5. Pour in the creamed cauliflower mixture and add the mushrooms and tremella extract. Simmer for 5 minutes more. Season with salt and pepper and serve immediately.

Notes • *Bone broth or chicken stock can be substituted for those who don't require a vegetarian version.*

Fresh tremella mushrooms can be hard to find but will also work.

Kale Salad with Mushroom "Croutons"

Paleo • Vegetarian • Gluten-free • Low-glycemic • Low-fat

Kale has had a big moment over the past few years, but any other dark, leafy green will work just as well in this recipe. They all have high concentrations of chlorophyll, which give them their characteristic deep green color. Chlorophyll also has antioxidant properties that prevent cell damage, promote cell healing, reduce inflammation, and aid with digestion, so it's safe to say that the more chlorophyll you consume, the better off you and your skin are.

Greens aside, what really sets this salad apart are the croutons. Most commercially available croutons are a nutritional wasteland with zero flavor, so for this dish, we've done a 'shroomy crouton redux. Their earthy, nutty flavor complements the bitterness of the kale, giving us good reason to get back on the kale train. Feel free to experiment with this recipe, adding your favorite seasonal vegetables to create your own perfect balance of crunch and flavor.

SERVES 2

TOTAL TIME: 10 MINUTES

10 ounces fresh shiitake mushrooms, cut into $1/2$-inch cubes

$1/2$ cup olive oil

2 tablespoons fresh lemon juice

Salt and freshly ground black pepper

1 pound kale or leafy green of your choice

3 tablespoons balsamic vinegar

3 ounces Parmesan cheese, shaved with a vegetable peeler

2 red onions, thinly sliced

5 tomatoes, cut into wedges

2 English cucumbers, sliced

½ cup pitted black olives, sliced

10 pepperoncini

1. Preheat the oven to 400°F. Line a baking sheet with parchment paper.
2. In a large bowl, toss the mushrooms with ¼ cup of the olive oil, the lemon juice, and salt and pepper to taste until they're evenly coated. Spread the mushrooms out evenly on the prepared baking sheet and bake for 15 minutes, stirring halfway through, until they are uniformly brown and crispy on the outside.
3. While the mushrooms are baking, place the kale in a large bowl and add the remaining ¼ cup olive oil, the vinegar, Parmesan, and onion. Massage the kale mixture with your hands until the leaves soften, 3 to 4 minutes.
4. Add the tomatoes, cucumbers, olives, and pepperoncini. Season with salt and pepper.
5. To serve, divide the salad between two plates and top with the hot, crispy shiitake mushroom "croutons."

RECIPES FOR
SPORTS PERFORMANCE

. . . .

All the medicinal and culinary mushrooms we highlight in this book are effective in terms of bringing oxygen to your cells, which will always make a noticeable impact on your energy levels. But none compare to cordyceps when it comes to providing significant, immediate boosts of energy. This fungus is basically a natural steroid. Cordyceps increases adenosine triphosphate (ATP) levels in the body and can seriously get you going (see more on page 48). So before you make any of the following recipes, it might be a good idea to lace up your sneakers.

Cordyceps Cubes with Coconut Water

Paleo • Vegan • Gluten-free • Low-fat

Sometimes when you need a quick jolt of energy, the act of even *acquiring* that energy can feel overwhelming. With this recipe, you can solve the problem before it becomes one because you'll have cubes of energy chilling in your freezer. I usually make a tray of these cubes, then store them in a freezer bag and keep the process going so I always have a supply ready to go. We made these cubes with coconut water because of its ability to replenish electrolytes and its incredible hydrating effects on the body. You can add these cubes to anything you're drinking, but they're especially good in coconut water because they won't dilute the beverage as they melt. Coconut water combined with the energetic powers of cordyceps makes these ice cubes the ideal addition to any preworkout drink.

MAKES 12 CUBES (2 OR 3 SERVINGS)

TOTAL TIME: 2 MINUTES PLUS OVERNIGHT FREEZING TIME

½ teaspoon potent cordyceps mushroom extract

2 cups coconut water, plus more for serving

1. In a measuring cup with a spout, stir the cordyceps extract into the coconut water until completely dissolved.
2. Pour the mixture into the wells of a 12-cube ice cube tray and freeze until solid, 8 to 12 hours.
3. To serve, add 4 to 6 cordyceps ice cubes to a glass of coconut water (or beverage of choice) and enjoy slowly, allowing the ice to fully melt into the drink.

Watermelon Cordyceps Energizer

Paleo • Vegan • Gluten-free • Low-fat

This drink is a super-hydrating (watermelon is over 90 percent water) energy booster. Watermelon also contains a substance called citrulline that has been known to alleviate muscle soreness due to its ability to improve and increase blood flow. Most of the citrulline in watermelon is concentrated in the rind, so we suggest adding as much of the white inner rind as you can to this drink. The natural sugars from the fruits combine with the chemical compounds in the cordyceps to keep you going throughout even the most rigorous of workouts. And as a bonus, we added a little ginger—thanks to its digestive properties, this won't sit in your stomach the way most sugary sports drinks do.

SERVES 2
TOTAL TIME: 10 MINUTES

½ small watermelon (about 5 cups)

½ pound strawberries, hulled

1 teaspoon (about 2 grams) cordyceps extract powder

1-inch piece ginger, peeled

10 ice cubes

Using a sharp knife, slice all the flesh, including a good bit of the white rind, from the watermelon skin. Add all the ingredients to a blender or Vitamix and blend on high for about 30 seconds, until smooth. Pour into glasses and serve.

Mushroom Hot Chocolate

Paleo • Vegetarian • Gluten-free

Who doesn't love the warm comfort that is a cup of hot chocolate? Incorporating mushrooms gives the drink some needed health benefits without compromising flavor. This is a fairly basic base recipe, and there are countless ways to customize your cacao. Add spices like cayenne or cinnamon, other superfoods like hemp and lucuma, flavors like vanilla and almond . . . and anything else you might fancy.

SERVES 2

TOTAL TIME: 5 MINUTES

- ½ cup cacao butter (see Note)
- 3 tablespoons unsweetened cacao powder (see Note)
- 2 tablespoons ghee
- 2 tablespoons coconut palm sugar (substitute xylitol for a sugar-free option)
- 2 teaspoons mushroom extract of choice (we recommend chaga, reishi, and cordyceps)
- ¼ cup raw cashews, soaked overnight
- ½ teaspoon pure vanilla extract
- Pinch of sea salt

Combine all the ingredients and 2 cups hot water in a high-speed blender. Blend on high for 15 to 30 seconds, until mixture becomes super creamy. Use caution when removing the blender lid, as the hot water will create *very* hot steam. Taste the hot chocolate, adding more mushroom extracts and cacao powder if you prefer your drink on the bitter side, or more sweetener if you prefer a more dessertlike drink.

Note • *In place of the cacao butter and cacao powder, you can instead use 2½ ounces of melted dark (70 to 80% cacao) chocolate.*

Superfood Sports Gel with Cordyceps and Beets

Paleo • Vegetarian • Gluten-free • Low-fat

Beets contain powerful chemical compounds called nitrates that convert to nitric oxide molecules in our bodies. Nitric oxide has been proven to increase blood flow by relaxing and expanding blood vessel walls, and it also increases oxygen usage on a cellular level. All that translates to an increase in physical stamina, which is key when it comes to athletic performance. Here, we've also added the superfood chia (whose fiber, good fats, and proteins also result in increased energy), cordyceps, honey, and salt. Think of the honey and salt as your workout bookends; the sugar in the honey provides that initial quick hit of energy while the salt replenishes any electrolytes lost during a vigorous workout. This is a go-go gel like no other.

MAKES 10 ENERGY SHOTS

TOTAL TIME: 30 MINUTES

2 red beets, peeled and chopped small

2 teaspoons chia seeds

2 tablespoons raw honey

2 teaspoons cordyceps extract powder

2 pinches of salt

1. Put the beets and 1 cup water in a small saucepan, cover, and bring to a boil. Cook the beets for 20 to 30 minutes, until they're very tender.
2. Discard the water and use an immersion blender to puree the cooked beets, then let cool to room temperature.
3. Once the beet puree has cooled, add the chia seeds, honey, cordyceps, and salt. Use the immersion blender to puree until the mixture reaches a gel-like consistency, adding water as needed. Add the

water little by little to find the right consistency, which can vary a bit with different chia seeds.

4. Store the gel in a sealed jar in the refrigerator for several weeks. Take a teaspoon or so whenever you need extra energy or before a workout.

Note • You can also portion the gel into mini sealable plastic bags to take with you on long runs, bike rides, or hikes. Just squeeze the gel directly into your mouth whenever you need a boost.

RECIPES FOR
BRAIN HEALTH

· ·

When it comes to your cognitive and neurological well-being, one mushroom rises above all the others. There is no question that lion's mane's powerful effects on brain function are extraordinary. Lion's mane not only offers protection from diseases like Alzheimer's, dementia, and Parkinson's, but it also can be extremely effective when it comes to general loss of brain function associated with aging or brain trauma, and even reverse cognitive deterioration. You probably never thought that eating pancakes and pie would make you smarter, but now with our mushroom-powered versions, they can. So go on . . . feed your head.

Wild Green Salad with Lion's Mane

Paleo • Vegan • Gluten-free • Low-glycemic • Low-fat

Walnuts, the top nut when it comes to brain health, work with lion's mane to give this salad its brain-boosting power. Walnuts contain plentiful amounts of omega-3 fatty acids, which have been shown to improve cognitive function and protect against cognitive decline (and they have a solid reputation for lowering blood pressure, too). We added sprouts for their brain-healthy vitamins and minerals and tomatoes for a dose of lycopene, an antioxidant that has been heavily studied as an effective combatant to cerebral decline. You'll get smart with this superfood salad, and it happens to taste super good, too.

SERVES 4 AS AN APPETIZER OR SIDE DISH

TOTAL TIME: 30 MINUTES

- 1 cup dandelion leaves, torn
- 1 cup chickweed, torn
- 1 cup lamb's quarter leaves, torn
- 1 cup purslane, torn
- 2 heads romaine lettuce, torn
- 3 tablespoons olive oil
- 2 tablespoons balsamic vinegar
- Salt
- 1 cup sprouts of your choice (sunflower, alfalfa, broccoli, etc.)
- 3 tomatoes, sliced
- ½ cup pitted kalamata or botija olives
- ½ cup whole walnuts, toasted
- 2 tablespoons butter or oil of your choice (we prefer ghee for this recipe)
- 6 ounces fresh lion's mane mushrooms, diced, or 2 cups dehydrated lion's mane, soaked for 2 hours, drained, and diced
- 1 medium onion, sliced
- Freshly ground white pepper

1. Mix together the wild greens and romaine lettuce in a large bowl.
2. In a small bowl or measuring cup, whisk together the olive oil, vinegar, and salt to taste until emulsified. Add to the greens and massage briefly with your hands.
3. Add the sprouts, tomatoes, olives, and walnuts and toss gently to combine. Refrigerate while you prepare the mushrooms to allow the flavors to meld.
4. In a skillet, melt the butter over medium heat. Add the mushrooms and onion and cook for about 10 minutes, until softened and slightly browned. Season with salt and white pepper.
5. To serve, divide the salad among four plates and top with the warm mushroom mixture.

What's in a Salad

We actually developed this dish after harvesting a pile of varied leafy greens while we were out foraging for mushrooms. If you have access to wild greens, it's a great idea to learn to identify the plants in your area, preferably with an experienced forager as a guide so you can make safe selections. Wild greens are much more nutritious than the cultivated greens you find in grocery stores. If you don't have the ability or inclination to forage, take a look at what's available at your grocer or farmers' market. While peppery greens like arugula work especially well in this recipe, any greens will do, and you might have fun swapping out more traditional greens in your other leafy meals. It's amazing how different layers of flavors will emerge depending on the bed they lie on.

Lion's Mane Pancakes

Paleo • Vegetarian • Gluten-free • Low-glycemic

With these healthier pancakes, you won't have to wait for a celebratory brunch or a snowy Sunday at home to dig in to a satisfying stack. Pancakes are first and foremost a comfort food, so we left in a lot of the good stuff like butter, eggs, and syrup. But since we're all about upping the healthy ante where we can, we snuck in some spinach and even give you an option to make these gluten-free. It's a good thing the lion's mane in these pancakes will help you think more clearly because you'll have some important decisions to make upon serving them: Syrup or jam? Juice or mimosa?

SERVES 5 (20 SMALL OR 5 LARGE PANCAKES)

TOTAL TIME: 30 MINUTES

3 large eggs

2 cups almond milk

1 cup packed fresh spinach, finely chopped

1 cup spelt flour (substitute cassava flour for gluten-free pancakes)

3 tablespoons unsalted butter, melted, plus more for cooking and serving

1 teaspoon salt

1 teaspoon freshly ground black pepper

8 ounces fresh lion's mane mushrooms (or 3 cups dehydrated lion's mane, soaked for 2 hours; see Note)

Jam or pure maple syrup, for serving (optional)

1. In a large bowl, vigorously whisk together the eggs and almond milk.
2. Add the spinach, flour, butter, salt, pepper, and mushrooms and stir until smooth. Let rest at room temperature for 15 minutes.
3. Set a cast-iron pan over high heat. When the pan is hot, add a liberal amount of butter and allow to melt. Add ½ cup of the pancake

batter to the pan. When little bubbles appear on the surface of the batter, use a spatula to check if the underside of the pancake is golden brown. If so, flip and fry on the other side for 1 to 2 minutes more. Repeat until all the batter has been used.

4. Serve hot with butter, jam, or syrup. Pancakes are also delicious eaten cold the next day. Store in a sealed container in the fridge overnight.

Note • *You can also try shiitake, oyster, or enoki mushrooms in this recipe.*

Key Lion's Mane Pie

Paleo • Vegan • Gluten-free

If you're one of the many people out there who are intimidated by the precision that traditional baking requires, you'll be excited to learn that this fun(guy) take on key lime pie requires zero baking skills. It's an icebox pie, so it's nearly impossible to mess up—it just needs to chill. And you can do the same, because this dessert has a two-ingredient crust and a filling that's as easy as . . . Well, you get the idea. The end result is sweet and tangy, a perfect summer dessert. Serve it the night before you have a big meeting; you're going to need that extra brainpower.

MAKES ONE 9-INCH ROUND PIE, TO SERVE 8 TO 10

TOTAL TIME: 30 MINUTES PREP TIME PLUS 2 HOURS FREEZING TIME

FOR THE CRUST
1 cup pitted dates, plus more if needed

1 cup raw walnuts, plus more if needed

FOR THE FILLING
1 cup cashews, soaked for at least 4 hours and drained

³/₄ cup canned coconut milk, well shaken

¹/₄ cup coconut oil, melted, plus more for greasing

5 grams lion's mane extract powder (about 1 heaping teaspoon)

Zest and juice of 8 key limes or use 4 Persian (standard) limes

¹/₂ cup raw honey

Pinch of salt

1. Lightly grease a 9-inch round springform pan with coconut oil. Line the bottom with parchment paper cut to fit and lightly grease the parchment.

2. To make the crust, in a food processor, pulse the dates until they are uniformly chopped but still a bit chunky. Transfer the dates to a bowl.

3. In the food processor, pulse the walnuts until they resemble a coarse meal (do not overprocess or they will turn into nut butter!). Return the dates to the food processor with the walnuts and process until a loose dough forms. If the dough does not come together into a loose ball, add a few more dates. If it seems *too* sticky, add a few more nuts. The dough should be tacky to the touch, but not fully stick to your fingers.

4. Press the dough into the bottom of the prepared pan. Place in the freezer to set as you prepare the filling.

5. To make the filling, combine all the filling ingredients in a high-speed blender and blend on high until creamy and smooth. Taste and adjust the flavor as needed, adding more lime juice or honey as desired.

6. Pour the filling over the chilled crust and freeze for 2 hours. Let sit at room temperature for 10 minutes before slicing and serving.

Reishi-Mucuna Lemonade

Paleo • Vegan • Gluten-free • Low-glycemic • Low-fat

Mucuna pruriens, which can be found in powdered form online or at most health stores, is often referred to as the "velvet bean." It's known in some circles for its effectiveness as an aphrodisiac, but our primary interest in mucuna is how it can positively affect your mood and cognitive function. Mucuna contains L-Dopa, an amino acid that converts to dopamine in the brain—meaning it can give you a happier outlook and increased brainpower. It has a sweet-smoky flavor, almost like burnt caramel, that contrasts nicely against the bittersweet lemonade and maple syrup. Chia will give you additional energy to keep you on your toes, while reishi will work its magic as the queen of medicinal mushrooms.

SERVES 4

TOTAL TIME: 15 MINUTES

2 tablespoons chia seeds

1 cup very strong reishi tea (see Notes), cooled to room temperature

1 teaspoon mucuna extract

Pinch of salt

¼ cup pure maple syrup

½ cup fresh lemon juice (from about 3 lemons)

1. In a measuring cup with a spout, stir the chia seeds into the reishi tea. Let them soak for about 10 minutes, stirring occasionally, until the seeds have absorbed the liquid and taken on a gel-like texture.
2. Stir in the mucuna and salt.
3. In a pitcher, mix together the maple syrup and lemon juice, stirring vigorously to dissolve the syrup. Add 2 cups cold water and stir to combine.

4. Pour the lemonade into four glasses and carefully pour the chia gel on top (see Notes). Serve with a straw.

Notes • *You can make reishi tea by cooking two or three pieces of reishi in very hot water for at least 30 minutes, or by mixing 1 teaspoon reishi extract/reishi elixir powder with hot water.*

If you're taking the lemonade to go, you can mix in the chia, but be mindful about how much you use, as it will absorb the liquid as it sits and you'll be left with gooey gel instead of a delicious drink.

MUSHROOM COFFEE RECIPES

. . . .

Though coffee culture has become ubiquitous, the consumption of coffee can be a remarkably complex, multifaceted experience, ranging from a mindless daily habit to a ritual of an almost spiritual nature. Depending on the day or hour, it can feel like a requirement, a reward, an opportunity to unwind, or a mandate to rev up. Coffee is a big deal, and I should know—we Finns drink on average a record number of 4 to 5 cups per day.

When you tell people you've taken to drinking mushroom coffee, the immediate reaction may be alarm mixed with a little bit of disdain. It's like saying you only drink decaf! But mushroom coffee is legitimately delicious, effective, and healthy stuff. You can still have your coffee—however you like it—but you won't experience the crash or jitters that accompany normal caffeine stimulation. Once you've become a bonafide mushroom coffee crusader (and you will), you'll be ready for the next-level coffee recipes in this section.

Chaga Un-Coffee

Paleo • Vegan • Gluten-free • Low-glycemic • Low-fat

Unlike the mushroom coffees we sell at Four Sigmatic, which do contain a microdose of coffee, this version is completely caffeine-free. Chaga has a flavor that is quite similar to coffee, making this drink a wonderful alternative for those who are very sensitive to caffeine in general or enjoy drinking coffee late in the afternoon or evening but then find that their sleep quality suffers. We've also added dandelion root here for its natural coffee-like taste and myriad health benefits, which include aiding in the elimination of bodily toxins, providing immune support, stabilizing blood sugar, and acting as a digestive aid. Mix that with chaga's many benefits, and you'll see how *un*believably good for you this *un*-coffee is.

MAKES 4 CUPS

TOTAL TIME: 5 MINUTES PLUS 4 HOURS BOILING TIME

> 2 tablespoons ground chaga
>
> 1 tablespoon roasted dandelion root (see sidebar)
>
> Finishing touches (nut milk, sweetener of choice, ground cinnamon, etc.)

1. In a saucepan, combine the chaga and about 4 cups water and bring to a boil. Boil for about 3 hours, continually adding water as it evaporates to maintain the water level (you want to have about 4 cups the entire time). Don't ever leave the saucepan unattended, as the water can evaporate quickly, and dry chaga can easily catch on fire.

2. After about 3 hours of boiling, add the roasted dandelion root to the saucepan. Boil for 1 hour more. Strain the coffee and divide it among four mugs. Serve hot, with the finishing touches you desire.

DANDELION ROOT HOW-TO

Roasted dandelion root can be found online at Amazon or at just about any natural health food store, but it's also easy to make your own. Here's how:

1. Dig up several bunches of dandelion roots. Dandelion is a common weed, so they should be fairly easy to find. They are best when harvested in early spring or late fall when the energy of the plant is mainly contained in the root as opposed to the parts aboveground, but dandelion harvested any time of year will work.

2. Wash the dandelion roots as well as you can, then chop them into medium-size pieces. Dry the chopped root in a dehydrator or toast in a 320°F oven for about 1 hour, or until fully dry.

3. Increase the oven temperature to 350°F and chop the root pieces into small dice. Return them to the baking sheet.

4. Toast for 30 to 40 minutes. Remove from the oven and let the root pieces cool slightly. Once they are cool enough to handle, use a spatula to press them against the pan into an even finer powder.

5. Place the powder back in the oven for 5 to 10 minutes. Remove from the oven and allow the powder to cool completely. Once cool, store the roasted dandelion root in an airtight container at room temperature, as you would store regular coffee.

Mushroom Butter Coffee

Paleo • Vegetarian • Gluten-free • Low-glycemic

If you didn't raise an eyebrow when you read "butter coffee," then you've been paying pretty close attention to recent food trends. Butter coffee has earned considerable media attention simply based on how bizarre it sounds. But when you consider that the good fats in butter, like its omega-3 and omega-6 fatty acids, can deliver sustained energy, and that butter's conjugated linoleic acid (CLA) has been shown to actually *reduce* body fat, butter coffee's trendiness is well deserved. Combining those buttery benefits with the immunomodulating and adaptogenic properties of mushrooms results in a health-boosted beverage like no other.

SERVES 4

TOTAL TIME: 5 MINUTES

4 cups prepared hot coffee

2 tablespoons unsalted butter or ghee

2 tablespoons coconut oil

$\frac{1}{2}$ teaspoon mushroom extract of your choice (lion's mane for brain power, cordyceps for energy, maitake for weight loss help, etc.)

Finishing touches (ground cinnamon, vanilla extract, unsweetened cacao powder, etc.; optional)

Combine the prepared coffee, butter, coconut oil, and mushroom extract in a high-speed blender and blend for 15 to 30 seconds. Be careful when opening the blender lid, as the steam will be very hot. Divide the coffee among four mugs and serve immediately. If you like, doctor up the coffee with the finishing touches of your choice.

Healthy Lion's Mane Latte

Paleo • Vegan • Gluten-free • Low-glycemic • Low-fat

We can all use a bit of a brain boost every now and then. The problem is that we normally can't simply order up these moments of brilliance—until now. Thanks to the lion's mane in this latte, you'll feel sharper and on your game. This drink is easier to make if you have an espresso machine, but we've designed it so you can make it without one as well. As far as the milk you choose, soy tends to foam up in the prettiest, silkiest manner, making it a good option for those who want to let their inner latte artist out. Almond is the trickiest for getting good, consistent foam, but mixing in a bit of coconut milk can help (and it's a delicious combo). Experimenting is encouraged . . . and it might be inevitable. After all, your brain will be working in overdrive after you've downed this drink.

SERVES 1

TOTAL TIME: 5 MINUTES

½ cup strong hot coffee (espresso is recommended, but use whatever you like)

½ teaspoon lion's mane extract

½ cup nondairy milk (soy, almond, cashew, coconut, hemp, etc.)

Dash of ground cinnamon

Dash of grated nutmeg

2 tablespoons whipped cream (optional)

1. In a mug, mix the lion's mane extract into the coffee.
2. Heat the milk using the steam wand on an espresso machine, until you reach your desired level of foam. You can also do this on the stovetop by shaking the milk carton vigorously before heating it in a small saucepan.

3. Pour the steamed milk into the mushroom coffee mix. Add the cinnamon, nutmeg, and whipped cream, if you like.

Note • *You can easily make this an iced latte by using cold milk and adding a few ice cubes to the finished drink.*

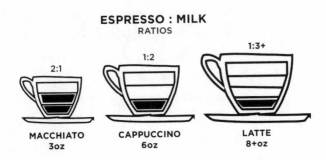

ESPRESSO : MILK
RATIOS

2:1

1:2

1:3+

MACCHIATO
3oz

CAPPUCCINO
6oz

LATTE
8+oz

Reishi Cappuccino

Paleo • Vegan • Gluten-free • Low-glycemic

Mushroom coffees are so fantastic because they don't require you to give up your beloved cup of joe, yet they eliminate some of the less-appealing effects caffeine can have on the body. In this cappuccino, reishi's adaptogenic properties support your hormonal system to prevent overstimulation, mitigating the jitters that straight-up coffee can create, and balance the coffee's acidity, making it easier on your digestive system. We've also added coconut butter and plant-based milk for some good fats and sustainable energy. The result is a calm, sustained focus, rather than a quick-hit, crazed rush. And it's smooth as silk to boot.

SERVES 1

TOTAL TIME: 10 MINUTES

1/2 cup prepared hot coffee (as strong as you like it)

1 teaspoon coconut butter

1/2 teaspoon reishi extract

1/2 cup rice or nut milk

Unsweetened cacao powder (optional)

Coconut palm sugar (optional)

1. While the coffee is still very hot, add the coconut butter and reishi extract and stir well to combine. Pour into a mug.
2. In a saucepan, heat the milk over medium heat. When it's fairly hot, whisk it vigorously (or use a milk frother) to create a silky foam.
3. Pour the foamy milk into the coffee, using a spoon to strain the solid milk in first and then top it off with a thick layer of foam. Top with a sprinkle of cacao powder and coconut sugar, if you like.

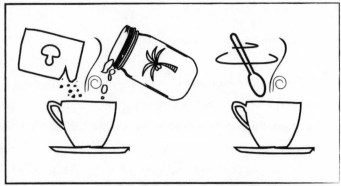

BREW THE COFFEE THE WAY YOU LIKE IT (ESPRESSO MACHINE, FRENCH PRESS, AEROPRESS, ETC.). WHILE COFFEE IS STILL VERY HOT, ADD COCONUT BUTTER AND REISHI EXTRACT AND STIR WELL TO COMPLETELY COMBINE. POUR INTO A MUG.

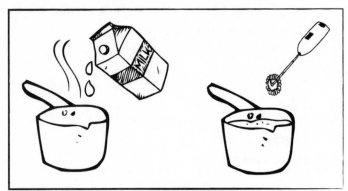

HEAT THE MILK IN A SAUCEPAN OVER MEDIUM HEAT (NO, USING A MICROWAVE IS NOT COOL). WHEN MILK IS FAIRLY HOT, WHISK IT BRISKLY (OR USE A MILK FROTHER) TO CREATE A NICE QUANTITY OF SILKY FOAM.

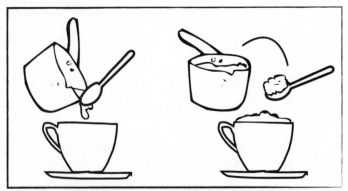

POUR HEATED MILK INTO THE COFFEE, USING A SPOON TO STRAIN THE SOLID MILK IN FIRST AND THEN TOPPING IT OFF WITH A THICK LAYER OF FOAM (SEE PICTURE). TOP WITH A SPRINKLE OF CACAO POWDER AND COCONUT SUGAR IF YOU LIKE.

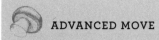 **ADVANCED MOVE**

If you want to boost your drink, consider adding ½ teaspoon ashwagandha, he shou wu, cistance, mucuna, or maca. Any of these powerful superfoods will give your reishi cappuccino additional hormonal support.

NEXT-LEVEL DESSERTS

· ·

When developing these dessert recipes, we wanted to strike a balance between "hiding" the mushrooms within these sweet treats and allowing them to shine as a featured component of the dish (just see page 170 for our recipe for ice cream with 'shroomy bits!). You don't *have* to tell your dinner guests that the super-dense chocolate cake they just enjoyed was packed with chaga, but why wouldn't you? People want to feel good about eating dessert, and now they can. You may want to wait until after they've scraped the last bit from their plate, just to enjoy the expressions on their faces when they learn they've been gobbling up mushrooms. Now *that's* dessert with double the satisfaction—we told you we'd deliver!

Cordyceps Raw Vegan Cheesecake

Paleo • Vegan • Gluten-free

When you hear the word *mushrooms*, the next word you think of probably isn't *romance*. But after you taste this dessert, it just might be. The delicate and creamy texture of this raw vegan cheesecake is utterly decadent. And since it's made with libido-enhancing cordyceps, this dessert is the perfect finish to any dinner *à deux*.

SERVES 10

TOTAL TIME: 30 MINUTES PLUS 4 HOURS CHILLING TIME

2 cups raw cashews

1 teaspoon sea salt

FOR THE BASE

½ cup raw almonds

½ cup pitted dates

2 teaspoons fresh lemon juice

1 tablespoon coconut oil, melted

Pinch of salt

FOR THE FILLING

½ cup pure maple syrup

½ cup coconut oil, melted

2 tablespoons fresh lemon juice

5 grams cordyceps extract powder (about 1 heaping teaspoon)

¼ cup coconut milk

¼ teaspoon pure vanilla extract

¼ teaspoon sea salt

1. Put the cashews in a medium bowl with 4 cups water and 1 teaspoon of the sea salt. Stir gently to combine and cover bowl with a thin tea towel. Set aside at room temperature for at least 2 hours.

2. To make the base, put the almonds and dates in the bowl of a food processor. Process until they form a uniform paste. Add the lemon juice, coconut oil, and salt and process until a loose dough forms.

3. Press the dough evenly into a 6- or 7-inch springform pan. Place in the freezer to set, about 2 hours.

4. Drain the cashews carefully and pat dry with paper towels.

5. To make the filling, in a blender, combine the cashews, maple syrup, coconut oil, lemon juice, cordyceps extract powder, coconut milk, vanilla, and salt. Blend on high for several minutes, until you obtain a completely smooth and creamy texture.

6. Pour the filling on top of the chilled base and refrigerate for about 2 hours to set. Let the cheesecake sit at room temperature for 10 minutes before slicing and serving.

Superfood Mudcake

Gluten-free

Rich chocolate desserts are always a crowd-pleaser, and this dense cake is no exception. It's super simple to make, and we guarantee that everyone will be asking for the recipe as they hold out their plate for a second serving. What really makes this dessert is the quality of the ingredients, so splurge on European-style butter and the best quality chocolate you can afford— you'll be glad you did. This recipe features chaga and superberries, which, when used together, can support eye and skin health. With generous quantities of butter, eggs, and cream, this cake isn't exactly light, but it's the perfect dessert for a day of celebration or a day of indulgence. It may not be low in calories, but its high amounts of nutrients more than make up for it.

SERVES 8

TOTAL TIME: 1 HOUR

Coconut oil for greasing

1 cup (2 sticks) unsalted butter

8 ounces dark chocolate (70 to 80% cacao), chopped

4 large eggs, lightly whisked

1 cup coconut palm sugar

$\frac{1}{2}$ cup maca powder

$\frac{1}{4}$ cup berry powder of choice (goji, bilberry, açai, etc.)

1 teaspoon chaga extract powder

1 teaspoon baking soda

Pinch of salt

$\frac{1}{4}$ cup heavy cream

1. Preheat the oven to 400°F. Lightly grease an 8-inch round spring-form pan with coconut oil, line the bottom with parchment paper cut to fit, and lightly grease the parchment.

2. In a double boiler, melt the butter and chocolate over low heat. Once completely melted and smooth, vigorously whisk in the eggs and coconut palm sugar until completely combined.

3. Add the maca, berry powder, chaga extract powder, baking soda, salt, and cream and whisk to combine.

4. Pour the batter into the prepared pan and bake for 40 minutes. Let cool slightly before slicing and serving.

Reishi Chocolate Drops

Paleo • Vegan • Gluten-free • Low-glycemic

These chocolate treats are raw, vegan, and good for you, too. Here we use reishi spores instead of an extract—reishi spores are one of the most potent superfoods in the world due to the high quantity of triterpenes they contain. The triterpenes give the spores their characteristic bitter flavor, but here, they blend perfectly with the sweetness of the chocolate so that only a delicious smoky, nutty flavor remains. Using coconut palm sugar and stevia lowers the glycemic load, but if you don't like the flavor of stevia, feel free to substitute honey or agave nectar. You can easily purchase reishi spores online (see our shopping guide on page 189).

MAKES ABOUT 24 PIECES

TOTAL TIME: 25 MINUTES PLUS 2 HOURS FREEZING TIME

> 1 cup chopped cocoa butter or white chocolate chunks
>
> 1 cup coconut oil
>
> 1 tablespoon reishi spores
>
> 1 tablespoon coconut palm sugar
>
> 1/2 teaspoon pure vanilla extract
>
> Pinch of sea salt
>
> 1 cup unsweetened cacao powder
>
> Liquid stevia
>
> Dried berries, nuts, or seeds (optional)

1. Put the cocoa butter in a double boiler set over low heat (the low heat is important for preserving the enzymes in the cocoa butter). When completely melted, add the coconut oil. Use a whisk or milk frother to combine vigorously until the fats are emulsified.

2. Add the reishi spores, sugar, vanilla, and salt. Whisk again to combine.

3. Using a sifter or strainer, slowly add the cacao powder until the mixture reaches the consistency of a thick cream. You may need a bit more or less cocoa powder, as you want a liquid chocolate mixture that is neither too thick nor too runny. Taste and add a few drops of liquid stevia as desired.

4. Pour the mixture into two ice cube trays or the wells of two mini muffin tins. Garnish with dried berries, nuts, or seeds, if desired. Freeze for 2 hours to harden. Enjoy them cold but not frozen—let them sit on the counter for 5 to 10 minutes before serving.

 ADVANCED MOVE

Try adding tocotrienols (see page 126) to make your raw chocolate creamier.

Paleo Ice Cream with Honeyed 'Shroomy Bits

Paleo • Gluten-free • Low-glycemic

Who doesn't love ice cream? We knew this recipe had to deliver the same rich, creamy decadence that you get when you dip your spoon into the real stuff. We went through a lot of trial and error before coming up with this foolproof version. Two hours is the optimal freezing time, but unlike with traditional ice cream, you don't want this version to sit in the freezer for longer than that, as ice crystals will form and the texture won't be nearly as dreamy. Though you won't taste the mushrooms or the raw egg yolks (yes, raw egg yolks are a must for this recipe) in the ice cream, you will be surprised to find out that the sweet buttery topping contains some serious mushroom goodness. We've never been in line at an ice cream shop and heard "'shroomy bits, please!" in between requests for sprinkles and nuts, but we're guessing that it's only a matter of time before we do.

SERVES 4

TOTAL TIME: 10 MINUTES PLUS 2 HOURS FREEZING TIME

5 tablespoons unsalted butter, at room temperature

¼ cup coconut oil, melted

2 large organic whole eggs

2 large organic egg yolks

2 tablespoons coconut palm sugar

¾ cup ice

½ teaspoon apple cider vinegar

20 drops liquid stevia

2 to 4 grams cordyceps, lion's mane, or other mild mushroom extract powder (about 1 teaspoon; see Note)

1 teaspoon matcha tea powder plus ½ teaspoon spirulina
(this creates a beautiful green color)

Seeds from 1 vanilla bean

½ teaspoon ground cardamom

½ teaspoon ground cinnamon

1 tablespoon unsweetened cacao powder

Fresh berries

Honeyed 'Shroomy Bits (recipe below)

1. Combine all the ingredients, including any additional flavors you want, in a high-speed blender. Blend on high for 30 seconds, or until the mixture is creamy and uniform in texture.

2. Pour the mixture into a mold or freezer-safe container and freeze for 2 hours. You can also make this in an ice cream machine if you have one (follow the manufacturer's instructions). The ice cream will keep for 2 to 3 months. Let it sit at room temperature for 10 minutes before serving, and then top with Honeyed 'Shroomy Bits.

Note • *You can substitute other mushroom powders, but be sure to select a mushroom with a mild flavor. Reishi and chaga are not recommended, as both are too bitter.*

Honeyed 'Shroomy Bits

1 teaspoon unsalted butter

1 teaspoon honey

4 shiitake mushrooms, stemmed and finely chopped (lion's mane also works well)

In a small saucepan, melt the butter and honey together over medium-high heat. Add the chopped mushrooms and cook, stirring, for about 5 minutes. Set aside to cool completely.

MIXIN' UP
THE MUSHROOMS

Every bartender likes to have a few tricks up his or her sleeve, and with these 'shroomy drinks, there are plenty of liquid punches to pull. Cocktails are made for experimentation, so think of these recipes as foundational guidelines and build from there. Just have fun and have at it. We could add a lot more information here, but we've just served up more than forty recipes and are in need of a cocktail. Cheers all around!

Cordysex on the Beach

Paleo • Vegan • Gluten-free • Low-fat

Somewhere along the way, this drink became something of a legend. Maybe because the play on words in the name is incredibly apt—you know by now that cordyceps can make people frisky. That said, proceed with caution.

MAKES 2 DRINKS
TOTAL TIME: 5 MINUTES

> 1 cup 100% cranberry juice
>
> 1 peach, pitted
>
> 1 orange or grapefruit, suprêmed (see Note)
>
> 2 grams cordyceps extract
>
> 1 to 3 ounces vodka (optional)
>
> 3 big ice cubes
>
> Orange slices, for garnish

Combine the cranberry juice, peach, orange, cordyceps, vodka (if using), and ¼ cup cold water in a blender and blend until smooth. Serve over ice in a highball glass and garnish with an orange slice.

Note • *To suprême a citrus fruit, trim off the top and bottom of the fruit with a sharp knife. Set the fruit on its end and slice away all the peel and white pith, following the curves of the fruit. Slice to the left and right of each membrane. The citrus wedges should come out easily.*

Kahlúa Mushroom Coffee

Vegan • Gluten-free • Low-glycemic • Low-fat

Were you thinking about a mushroom Mudslide? Well, consider this your hot answer to that crazy frosty cocktail phenomenon of the nineties. Add a splash of nut milk if you really want to get wild.

MAKES 1 DRINK

TOTAL TIME: 5 MINUTES

- 1 teaspoon chaga, reishi, or cordyceps extract powder
- 1 cup prepared black coffee, hot
- 1 ounce Kahlúa liqueur

In a large mug, dissolve the mushroom powder into the hot coffee. Stir in the Kahlúa and serve.

Mulled Mushroom Wine

Paleo • Vegan* • Gluten-free • Low-fat

Mulled wine is an aromatic and comforting European winter tradition. We've added some 'shroomy goodness to further alleviate any wintertime blues.

SERVES 4

TOTAL TIME: 15 MINUTES

2 cups 100% apple juice

2 cups rich, full-bodied red wine (about ½ bottle)

1 teaspoon chaga extract

Zest and juice of 1 orange

3 whole cloves

1 cinnamon stick

4 allspice berries

Honey (optional)

In a medium saucepan, combine all the ingredients except the honey; heat over medium heat until just beginning to simmer (do not bring to a full boil or the alcohol will quickly burn off). Reduce the heat to low and simmer for 10 minutes. Strain the wine into cups and sweeten with a bit of honey, if desired. (If you do decide to use honey, then the recipe will no longer be vegan.)

Mushroom Chocolate Eggnog

Paleo • Vegetarian • Gluten-free • Low-fat

We've taken traditional 'nog and upped the ante with chocolate, brandy, and cordyceps. Grab a mug and hang out under the mistletoe.

MAKES 1 DRINK

TOTAL TIME: 10 MINUTES

- ½ cup prepared eggnog made with almond milk or coconut milk
- 1 teaspoon unsweetened cacao powder
- 1 teaspoon coconut palm sugar
- 1 teaspoon cordyceps extract powder
- ½ ounce brandy (optional)

Heat the eggnog in a small saucepan. Pour into a small mug and stir in the cacao powder, coconut palm sugar, and cordyceps mushroom extract. Add a dash of brandy, if desired.

Lion's Mane Whiskey

Paleo • Vegan • Gluten-free • Low-glycemic • Low-fat

It's said that a stiff drink can be a medicinal miracle, but we've never been sure if that was actually true or just wishful thinking. This drink, on the other hand, is guaranteed to make you feel better and think smarter.

MAKES 2 DRINKS

TOTAL TIME: 50 MINUTES

1 cup coarsely chopped dried lion's mane mushrooms

2 star anise pods

10 fresh mint leaves

5 to 10 drops liquid stevia

10 ice cubes

1 ounce high-quality grain-free whiskey

1. Bring 2 cups water to a boil in a medium saucepan. Add the mushrooms, star anise, and mint. Cover and boil for 10 minutes.
2. Remove the saucepan from the heat and let the "mushroom tea" steep for 20 minutes.
3. Strain the tea into two serving glasses and refrigerate for 20 minutes to cool.
4. When ready to serve, divide the stevia, ice cubes, and whiskey between the glasses.

MUSHROOM COMFORT FOOD

The dishes we include here are good gateway recipes to the mushroom world if you are feeling a bit hesitant about jumping into your funguy shoes and taking off at full speed. They're also great for kids—to help you both make and eat! Pizza, fries, dip, and cheesy, melty goodness are foods most of us can get on board with, so we've taken these comfort favorites and given them a 'shroomy twist. They're not meant to taste the same as their traditional versions, but we'd argue that they taste a lot better. Either way, the result will be the same: complete satisfaction.

Enoki Mushroom Fries

Paleo • Vegetarian • Gluten-free • Low-glycemic

We can't think of a better way to get the kids interested in mushrooms than by tempting them with a plate of fungi fries. However, we don't recommend that children participate in the actual cooking process here. Hot oil has a tendency to splatter, so this recipe needs to be closely monitored. If you want to cook with the kids, have them prepare the Mushroom Garlic Dip as an alternative to ketchup; it's delicious with the enoki fries. Though we call for beer in the batter, it's a minimal amount, and the alcohol will burn off as the fries cook—but if you want to keep this recipe 100 percent child-friendly, you're welcome to substitute another carbonated beverage. These mushroom fries aren't going to fool anyone as a French fry substitute, but their earthy, nutty taste—combined with their crisp-on-the-outside-and-soft-on-the-inside texture—make them just as craveable.

SERVES 4

TOTAL TIME: 30 MINUTES

¼ cup cornstarch

¼ cup coconut flour (or flour of your choice)

½ teaspoon baking powder

1 teaspoon ground turmeric

½ teaspoon ground cumin

1 large egg

¼ cup beer, kombucha, or other carbonated beverage

1 cup frying oil (we like to use a combination of equal parts grapeseed oil and ghee)

2 cups enoki mushrooms

Salt

Handful of fresh herbs, chopped (oregano, thyme, dill, etc.—use what you like!)

1. In a large bowl, whisk together the cornstarch, flour, baking powder, turmeric, and cumin. Beat in the egg and beer. You want the batter to be thick, but still "dippable," so add more liquid if needed.
2. In a large wok, stockpot, Dutch oven, or deep fryer, heat the oil to 325°F. Adjust the heat to maintain the temperature.
3. Coat the mushrooms in the batter, dipping and turning them in the bowl. Gently and carefully drop a handful at a time into the hot oil. Fry, flipping occasionally, until the mushroom fries are a deep golden-brown color and crisp all over, 4 to 6 minutes total. Transfer to a paper towel–lined plate to drain and sprinkle with salt. Repeat with the remaining mushrooms.
4. Transfer to a large serving plate. Sprinkle with fresh herbs and serve with Mushroom Garlic Dip (page 182) or ketchup.

Mushroom Garlic Dip

Vegetarian • Gluten-free • Low-glycemic

This simple dip is so versatile that you'll find yourself making it all the time. You can throw it together in minutes and serve with crudités as an after-school snack or last-minute dinner party appetizer. Leftovers make a great sandwich spread or toast topper. Feel free to play with the recipe and add spices and herbs as you like.

SERVES 4

TOTAL TIME: 5 MINUTES

2 garlic cloves, finely chopped

1 cup Greek yogurt

2 teaspoons fresh lemon juice

1 teaspoon turkey tail extract powder

Salt and freshly ground black pepper

In a small bowl, thoroughly mix together the garlic, yogurt, lemon juice, and mushroom extract powder. Season with salt and pepper. Serve with Enoki Mushroom Fries (page 180) or sliced veggies.

Raw Pizza

Paleo • Vegan • Gluten-free • Low-glycemic • Low-fat

Who doesn't love pizza? While we're never going to give up the real deal, we tend to crave it more often than we should be eating it (let's face it: pizza is a pretty hard sell on the health food front). We came up with this raw version as a worthy alternative so you can feel good about feeding your kids—and yourself!—this 'za as often as you like. With a slightly sweet, veggie-loaded crust, a twist on traditional tomato sauce, mock cheese, and marinated vegetable toppings, this rendition has earned a reputation as an unexpected crowd-pleaser.

The pizzas take a bit of preplanning, as the crust requires about 12 hours of dehydrating time. Preparing it with kids makes for a fun family activity—after all that waiting time, everyone will be eager to dig into the final dish.

MAKES 10 PIZZA ROUNDS

TOTAL TIME: 45 MINUTES ACTIVE PLUS DEHYDRATING TIME (10 TO 12 HOURS)

FOR THE CRUST
1 medium head cauliflower, chopped into florets

2 garlic cloves, coarsely chopped

¼ cup walnuts, coarsely chopped

2 tomatoes, coarsely chopped

1 small onion, coarsely chopped

2 tablespoons fresh lemon juice

3 fresh dates, pitted and coarsely chopped

1 teaspoon dried oregano

1 teaspoon salt

½ teaspoon freshly ground black pepper

FOR THE SAUCE

½ cup sun-dried tomatoes, soaked in water for 1 hour and drained

½ cup walnuts

½ bell pepper, coarsely chopped

3 fresh dates, pitted

2 small onions, coarsely chopped

1 tablespoon fresh lemon juice

1 tablespoon olive oil

1 tablespoon soy sauce

1 cup chopped shiitake, oyster, or enoki mushrooms (optional)

FOR THE MOCK CHEESE

½ cup tahini

3 tablespoons miso paste

2 tablespoons lecithin powder (see Note)

FOR THE PIZZA TOPPINGS

2 tablespoons apple cider vinegar

1 tablespoon soy sauce

1 tablespoon raw honey

3 ounces fresh shiitake mushrooms, stemmed and thinly sliced

2 onions, thinly sliced

½ bell pepper, thinly sliced

Fresh basil leaves, for garnish

1. Preheat the oven to 150°F (or the lowest temperature possible—we are shooting for around 115°F; alternatively, use a dehydrator). Position the racks in the upper and lower thirds of the oven and keep the door open slightly by wedging in a wooden spoon. This will lower the temperature slightly. Line two baking sheets with parchment paper.

2. In a food processor, pulse the cauliflower florets until evenly broken down into fine crumbles, then transfer to a large bowl.

3. In a high-speed blender, combine the garlic, walnuts, tomatoes, onion, lemon juice, dates, oregano, salt, and pepper and puree on high speed until smooth, 30 to 40 seconds. Add the puree to the bowl with the cauliflower and mix to combine.

4. Use your hands to shape the cauliflower mixture into ½-inch-thick, 5-inch diameter circles and place them on the prepared baking sheets.

5. Dehydrate in the oven for 5 to 6 hours, until the dough is solidified but not dry. Flip the circles and dehydrate for 5 to 6 hours more. The crusts are best consumed immediately, but they will keep, tightly wrapped and refrigerated, for up to 5 days or in the freezer for several months.

6. To make the sauce, combine all the sauce ingredients in the blender and blend on high until smooth, about 45 seconds. If the sauce looks too thick, add a bit of water to achieve the desired consistency. Store in an airtight container in the refrigerator until ready to use. The sauce can be made up to 1 week in advance.

7. To make the mock cheese, combine all the mock cheese ingredients and a dash of water in the blender and blend on medium speed until smooth, about 30 seconds. Store in an airtight container in the refrigerator until ready to use. The cheese can be made up to 1 week in advance.

8. For the pizza toppings, in a medium bowl, whisk together the vinegar, soy sauce, and honey. Add the mushrooms, onions, and bell pepper to the bowl and massage gently with your hands until evenly mixed. Let the veggies marinate in the refrigerator for 2 to 3 hours to soften.

9. To assemble the pizzas, place the crusts on a serving platter or plate

and spread the tomato sauce on top. Grate the cheese and sprinkle it evenly over each crust. Top with the marinated veggies and garnish with fresh basil leaves.

Note • *Lecithin powder is a soy- or sunflower-based emulsifier that will give the mock cheese a cheesy texture and nice flavor. You can find it online and at some natural foods stores and gourmet grocers.*

Stuffed Bell Peppers with Maitake

Vegetarian • Gluten-free • Low-glycemic

These stuffed peppers are such great comfort food. Warm, with melted cheese and a dollop of sour cream, they're the funguy alternative to a loaded baked potato—only a lot healthier and with much more flavor. Using a bit of butter gives the dish richness and the meaty maitake makes it satisfying and filling. Kids love anything with melted cheese (ahem, we *all* love anything with melted cheese), so here's another good way to get the younger ones excited about eating their vegetables.

SERVES 2

TOTAL TIME: 45 MINUTES

1 tablespoon unsalted butter or coconut oil

½ medium white onion, diced

½ cup brown rice

2 cups sliced maitake mushrooms

Juice of ½ lemon

1 small bunch flat-leaf parsley, chopped

1 teaspoon salt

2 large red bell peppers, halved crosswise, seeded, and rinsed

¼ cup shredded cheddar cheese

Sour cream, for serving (optional)

1. Preheat the oven to 400°F.
2. In a medium skillet, melt the butter over medium heat. Add the onion and cook, stirring, until tender and translucent, 3 to 5 minutes.
3. Add the rice and ¾ cup water to the skillet. Bring to a simmer and cook for about 10 minutes, or until most of the water has been absorbed by the rice.

4. Add the maitake, lemon juice, parsley, and salt and stir to combine. Cook for 5 minutes more.

5. Remove the mushroom-rice mixture from the heat and divide it evenly among the bell pepper halves. Sprinkle the tops with the cheese.

6. Stand the stuffed peppers upright on a baking sheet or in a baking dish and bake for 20 minutes, until the cheese has melted and the peppers have softened. Top each with a dollop of sour cream, if desired, and serve immediately.

5

SHOPPING GUIDE

Now that you know what mushrooms can do for your health and overall wellness, you're going to want to get your hands on some fungi . . . fast. We know not everyone lives near a Chinatown or a burgeoning farm or foraging scene (though fortunately, more and more locations have both of those things), but you can purchase mushrooms from a local mycologist, natural food store, or online. What matters most is quality. That said, it's important to know that there are few regulations on what can be considered a "mushroom" product, meaning that what you think you are getting could be vastly different from what you're actually getting. It's important to educate yourself a bit before purchasing, because, as with anything, "buyer beware" applies.

But we're here to help you, so don't worry too much—we've designed this section to ensure you find the best quality products possible. What we've chosen to include on this list is hardly exhaustive—new companies and products are popping up all the time and the market is rife with reliable, reputable sources. Unfortunately, it's also filled with products that are essentially completely ineffective. Pretty packaging and a good marketing strategy means that many subpar mushroom products are being purchased by people who are then left wondering why their expensive supplements seem to be doing nothing for them. We've been that person, and we're here to make sure that you never are.

What to Look for When Buying Mushroom Products

You could spend all day reading labels or diving down the rabbit hole of consumer reviews on each and every product you consider, but you don't need to make it that hard on yourself. Instead, we've broken down the buying process into four digestible parts:

1. DO THE DUAL

Remember the importance of dual-extraction from chapter 1. Mushrooms contain both water-soluble and fat-soluble compounds, and each plays an integral role in delivering the health benefits of medicinal mushrooms to your body. Both compounds need to be drawn out of the mushroom's fruiting body through a hot water and alcohol extraction process to ensure that you get the maximum amount of nutrition and health benefits possible. Whenever you purchase mushroom products, make sure that the labeling clearly states that the mushrooms were dual-extracted.

2. PICK THE FRUIT

While all parts of the mushroom play an important role in nature, the fruiting body is what delivers nutrients and healing benefits directly to humans. The fruiting body is what humans and animals have always eaten, as it's what is naturally available. As you begin researching different mushroom products, you'll notice that many of them are mycelium-based. These are less effective in terms of delivering health benefits than those that are fruiting-body-based, as the fruiting bodies can be extracted and concentrated much more readily than mycelium can.

Why is this? Mycelium is commercially grown on grains (usually rice), and when "mushroom" products are produced, the mycelium *and* the grain are ground together into a powder. This means that high amounts of the growing substrate and starch (additives that mushrooms don't naturally contain) are included in the final product. Mycelium products grown on grain are actually more akin to soy-fermented grain products—like tempeh, for example—than they are to real mushroom products. Always check how the mushroom product is derived and, if it does contain mycelium, how the mycelium is grown.

3. QUALITY CONTROL

Mushrooms have the ability to clean and purify our environment. They are the vacuum cleaners of the forest, so it makes sense that they can accumulate heavy metals, radiation, and certain pesticides along the way. Some mushrooms, even though they're antifungal agents, can collect harmful molds on their surfaces. Aim to find brands and products that have been tested against pesticides (even if they are certified organic), heavy metals, irradiation, and mycotoxins. This applies to both cultivated and wildcrafted mushrooms.

4. YOUR DAILY DOSE

While consuming any amount of the fungi's fruiting body is good for you, the efficacy is really only proven when you are getting adequate amounts of the active ingredients. A good rule of thumb is to use medicinal mushroom extracts with at least 20 percent polysaccharide content, so be sure that the products you purchase state as such. Then it's up to you to regulate how much you consume on a daily basis—500 to 2,000 mg is the optimal amount per dose (see the dosage chart on page 37).

Keep in mind that encapsulating mushroom powders usually requires adding fillers and lubricants—undesirable ingredients that provide no benefits to consumers but help machines make the capsules faster. When mushroom extract powders are loosely packed into individual packages, it eliminates the need for any fillers or additives. Don't get us wrong, mushroom capsules can be very effective, but adding mushroom powders to liquids ensures a more potent and efficient delivery of nutrients to your body.

Local Sourcing

If you find a local forager, don't be afraid to ask if you can join on an upcoming day trip—foragers are friendly folks in our experience.

1. CHINATOWN

If you're fortunate enough to live near a bustling Chinatown, then you're fungi fortunate indeed. Because medicinal mushrooms have been used in traditional Chinese medicine for centuries, start a conversation with a pharmacist in Chinatown and things will take off from there. For your next stop, you'll want to look to where the locals are shopping, as that's usually the most foolproof (not to mention easiest) way to spot a reputable seller for popular edible mushrooms like shiitake and inedible mushrooms like reishi. Many of the pharmacists and natural foods proprietors buy from the same suppliers, so you can be sure you'll get quality products no matter where you shop in Chinatown.

2. FARMERS' MARKET

Farmers' markets are another fruitful source for mushrooms, not only for edible (and sometimes even inedible) varieties, but also as a foraging networking arena. If none of the vendors have a bounty of mushrooms available, ask around to see who might be the area's foremost mushroom forager. You'll likely walk away with a name or two and will then be on your way to having your very own local mushroom source.

3. NATURAL FOOD STORES

At Whole Foods and other health food stores, you should be able to find fresh mushrooms like shiitake, enoki, oyster, and maitake. You may even see some lion's mane on store shelves from time to time, depending on your location. Don't be afraid to ask the owner of your local natural grocer to stock a good variety of mushrooms whenever possible. But know that many grocery store owners have optimized their facilities for plants and are often not very mushroom savvy, so you may need to be an educator as well as a consumer. No matter where you buy your mushrooms, give them a thorough once-over, checking for any molds that may have grown due to poor storage methods. You can cut off any affected areas, but sometimes that is not enough to get rid of all the mold. To be on the safe side, simply toss these mushrooms into your compost bin.

Surfing for 'Shrooms

Performing a web search for mushroom supplements is an exercise in information overload. So start with the places we recommend here and your base for reputable virtual sources will grow in no time. The funguy network is a tight one.

- *foursigmatic.com* offers the highest quality prepackaged mushroom drinks in the form of coffees, hot chocolates, lemonades, and a variety of other superfood blends.

- *mountainroseherbs.com* is one of the best online sources for purchasing natural products, like chaga, reishi, and shiitake in bulk. Their powdered cordyceps is also very reliable.
- *mushroomscience.com* and *mushroomwisdom.com* are two excellent sources for mushroom capsules, as they contain minimal fillers and are extracted from mushroom fruiting bodies.
- *rebeltonics.com* makes premade mushroom drinks for those who like their mushroom goodness delivered via tasty beverages. They are readily available nationwide.

Bonus: Be sure to check out our online guide to mushroom-friendly restaurants in cities like San Francisco, New York, and Los Angeles. Chefs are fungi fanatics!

FINAL WORDS

By now you probably know more about mushrooms and fungi than you thought you ever would, or maybe you feel like we've merely cracked open a door into a world that you will continue to explore in the weeks, months, and years to come. I hope the latter is the case, as there is so much more to learn and so many incredible benefits yet to be realized from the fungi kingdom. Whatever your stance, I look forward to hearing how the mushrooms we've focused on positively affect your life, as I have no doubt of their powers—let us know about your experiences through social media or via e-mail!

It's a true shame that mushrooms have not been on the forefront of most people's minds as a powerful healing tool. It's understandable, considering that, except for maybe a recent interest in chaga, prominent media outlets aren't yet touting their benefits. I'm confident that this will change soon—and you'll be ahead of the curve, maybe even becoming an effective mushroom crusader yourself. While Western cultures have traditionally been apprehensive about the efficacy of natural health and holistic healing, now, more than ever, we need as much support and as many resources as possible to take care of our overall well-being. The beneficial role mushrooms can play on our health and wellness is truly limitless.

Perhaps it's because of my childhood spent on a farm or my country's appreciation for nature and the wilderness, but my feeling is that life is a precious, precarious thing. It should be honored, but it's something you need to take upon yourself to bestow. It is up to you to act, take preventative measures, and protect yourself, whether physically, mentally, emotionally, or all of the above. Unfortunately, the chance that you will at some point be negatively affected by illness, environmental toxins and pollutants, hormonal imbalances, and other disease is pretty much inevitable. So when your health is concerned, don't be reactive. Be proactive.

We have a mind-set in Finland that we call *sisu*. While Finns are infamous for being insecure about their place in the world and their culture in general, *sisu* is representative of how we, as a nation, have historically been able to succeed even under the most unlikely circumstances. We have done this because we don't give up. Because we have guts. Because we demonstrate determination, resilience, and persistence. I mention this because I believe that mushrooms exemplify *sisu*. They have the relentless tenacity and strength needed to ward off unwanted bodily invaders. They have the ever-evolving capacity to adapt to unexpected circumstances and restore balance. Their abilities to help the body achieve optimal health and wellness, even when the odds are stacked against them, are limitless. It's impossible to truly quantify the myriad ways mushrooms can positively impact your life, yet they're capable of doing all these things and so much more. Quietly, persistently, and effectively.

You've met ten medicinal mushrooms that have the capacity to change your life, and now you have the vocabulary to discuss and understand the fungi kingdom as it becomes an increasingly prevalent health tool in our society. You can surprise your family and friends with the news that the chocolate cake they just gobbled up is loaded with powerful mushrooms, and maybe you'll even make some sauerkraut on your next date. You know where to source quality 'shroomy products, and you might soon replace your morning joe with mushroom coffee. So welcome to the club—you're now a funguy yourself!

And if you still have any doubts, let me close off with this: Santa Claus was a mushroom dealer. Yes, that jolly old fella was a big-time funguy. But that's a story for another time, perhaps best told over a cup of hot chaga tea.

AFTERWORD

Recently, adaptogenic mushrooms have become a big topic of research in the West. We're finding that certain varieties have exceptional medicinal properties and we're just scratching the surface. As we hit the limits of Western drug therapies, we're learning that the functional properties of these adaptogenic fungi are helping solve some of the modern lifestyle issues we're now encountering.

As a doctor of Oriental medicine, I've known of the amazing healing properties of adaptogenic mushrooms. I've used them for years with patients, corporate executives, and athletes. As a CEO and a family man, I use them to keep my own vitality up and help me lengthen my fuse in an increasingly complex and toxic world.

These mushrooms have long been revered by traditional healers, both past and present. My relationship with these mushrooms began through my studies of scholarly texts. The great Shennong spoke of the immense value of Reishi thousands of years ago, but we can't solely rely on these books anymore. We are in uncharted territory and have to deal with new modern-day challenges.

The ancient books talk about mushrooms' medicinal properties but actually understanding how to apply them to your daily life in today's age requires something special—*direct transmission*. We need to be shown firsthand how these mushrooms can work for us.

This is where Tero comes in. He is a rare type of person; with his extensive farming and wildcrafting background, he has dedicated his life to studying the link between health and mushrooms. He can walk you through a pine forest and find mushrooms with the skill of expert foragers of the past, but he also knows the science behind *why* these mushrooms work the way they do. He's a data-driven guy and a model for the herbalists of the future. Scientifically inquisitive and inspired by ancient wisdom, Tero represents the best of old and new, East and West.

With Tero as our guide, there's never been a better opportunity to preserve this tradition of using mushrooms for health and lean into learning all we can. The ancients have handed down immense knowledge and we now have incredible opportunities to apply our scientific curiosity to mushrooms and their role in our wellness.

Take the wisdom in this book to heart and use it in your life. Unlike with harsh medications, don't expect changes to take place overnight. With some patience, you'll slowly notice several improvements in your life. Things will start to go right. You'll have more enthusiasm, better immunity, increased stamina, and mental clarity. The body needs some time to recover before it can thrive, and these mushrooms are the secret ingredient. Once you bring them into your life, you'll never look back.

To your health,
Dr. Pedram Shojai
Founder of Well.Org
Producer of Vitality, Origins, and Prosperity
Author of *Rise and Shine*, *The Urban Monk*,
and *The Art of Stopping Time*

ACKNOWLEDGMENTS

I wish to thank the following people for helping to make this book a reality:

My mother, Pirkko, for taking me foraging at an early age and teaching me amazing things about nutrition and physiology;

My father, Markku, and my brother, Vesa, for their love, wisdom, and patience;

All my fellow funguys and fun-gals at Four Sigmatic. You've made this new journey so much fun. Special thanks to Markus Karjalainen, Juho Heinola, and Lari Laurikkala for helping with the photography, illustrations, and recipes, respectively;

My bank balance and former employers for providing me with the financial resources needed to be able to spend so many years working for mushrooms as an unpaid intern;

Pam Krauss, Nina Caldas, and everybody at Penguin Random House for giving me the opportunity to write this book;

Coleen O'Shea, Maggie White, and Nikki Van Noy for your professional support and guidance on turning a regular Finnish funguy into a published author;

All the world's mycologists and mushroom enthusiasts who walked before me.

I also want to thank every mushroom hater I've come across over the years for motivating me to write this book. Except for that one New York City Parks & Recreation employee who yelled at me for foraging mushrooms and told me that I would die if I ate them.

There are so many amazing people that deserve my gratitude, but to save space and your time I will stop here, and thank them in person.

Lari Laurikkala

My biggest gratitude always goes to Mother Nature. Special thanks to Mom, Dad, and my grandparents who guided me on my path to cherish nature and always took me mushroom foraging. Thanks to the whole Four Sigmatic gang, my muse Carly, our Holmenkollen-tribe in Finland, and all my other dear friends who have always inspired me to create something new and exciting in the kitchen. Because of you, we've been able to celebrate life together over nourishing meals countless times.

INDEX

athletic performance *(Cont.)*
    Superfood Sports Gel with Cordyceps
        and Beets, 141–42
    Watermelon Cordyceps Energizer, 139
avocados, *in* Chocolate-Avocado Mousse
    with Turkey Tail, 94–95

"Bacon," Mushroom, Broccoli Soup with,
    118–19
beauty aids
    Berry Blast Smoothie, 130–31
    chaga, 45
    Chaga Jelly Bowl, 120–21
    Chaga Skin Cream, 128
    enoki, 62
    Kale Salad with Mushroom
        "Croutons," 134–35
    oyster mushroom, 66
    shiitake, 54, 55
    shisandra, 131
    tremella, 67–69
    Vegetarian "Clam" Chowder, 132–33
Beets, Superfood Sports Gel with
    Cordyceps and, 141–42
Bell Peppers with Maitake, Stuffed,
    187–88
berries
    Berry Blast Smoothie, 130–31
    shisandra, 131
    Watermelon Cordyceps Energizer, 139
    beta-glucans, 22–23
beverages. *See also* cocktails; coffee
    Berry Blast Smoothie, 130–31
    Chaga Chai, 88–89
    Chaga Decoction, aka 'Shroom Tea,
        74–75
    Cordyceps Cubes with Coconut
        Water, 138
    Mushroom Hot Chocolate, 140
    Mushroom Jun Tea, 106–7
    Reishi Kombucha, 103–5
    Reishi-Mucuna Lemonade, 150–51
    reishi tea, 151
    Superfood Slushie, 114
    Turkey Tail Carob Elixir, 110–11
    Watermelon Cordyceps Energizer, 139
blood sugar regulation
    enoki for, 63
    ghee for, 80
    maitake for, 7, 20, 57
    Maitake Muffins, 84–85
    Oyster Mushroom Wild Rice Salad,
        78–79

Raw Vegan Sushi with Shiitake, 81–82
reishi for, 40
Shiitake Carpaccio, 83
brain function
    Healthy Lion's Mane Latte, 157–58
    Key Lion's Mane Pie, 148–49
    lion's mane for, 51–52, 143
    Lion's Mane Pancakes, 146–47
    Reishi-Mucuna Lemonade, 150–51
    Wild Green Salad with Lion's Mane,
        144–45
breads
    Lion's Mane Pancakes, 146–47
    Maca-Mushroom Buns, 115–16
    Maitake Muffins, 84–85
Broccoli Soup with Mushroom "Bacon,"
    118–19
Buns, Maca-Mushroom, 115–16
Butter Coffee, Mushroom, 156

cabbage, *in* Mushroom Sauerkraut,
    100–102
cacao. *See* chocolate
cancer. *See* anticancer agents
Cappuccino, Reishi, 159–61
carbohydrates, 20–21, 77
cardiovascular health, 54–55
Carob Turkey Tail Elixir, 110–11
Carpaccio, Shiitake, 83
cashews
    Broccoli Soup with Mushroom
        "Bacon," 118–19
    Cordyceps Raw Vegan Cheesecake,
        164–65
    Key Lion's Mane Pie, 148–49
    Mushroom Hot Chocolate, 140
cauliflower
    Raw Pizza, 183–86
    Raw Vegan Sushi with Shiitake, 81–82
    Vegetarian "Clam" Chowder, 132–33
chaga
    about, 43–46
    Chaga Chai, 88–89
    Chaga Decoction, aka 'Shroom Tea,
        74–75
    Chaga Jelly Bowl, 120–21
    Chaga Skin Cream, 128
    Chaga Un-Coffee, 154
    Kahlúa Mushroom Coffee, 175
    Miso Mushroom Seaweed Soup,
        98–99
    Mulled Mushroom Wine, 176
    Mushroom Hot Chocolate, 140

AUTHOR BIOS/COMPANY INFO

Tero Isokauppila

Growing up on his family's farm in Finland, Tero formed a keen interest in food, farming, and healing early in his life. He earned a degree in chemistry and a certificate in plant-based nutrition at Cornell University, and won a Finnish innovation award for his idea to export the culinarily coveted matsutake mushroom to Japan along the way. After living in eight countries on three continents, Tero has seen the astounding impact that health and wellness can have on individuals, communities, and the world at large. This understanding inspired him to found Four Sigmatic in 2012. Today, Tero is a sought-after subject-matter expert on all things pertaining to mushrooms, superfoods, and natural health, and has been a featured speaker at Summit Series, Wanderlust, WME-IMG, and Soho House. He was also chosen as one of the world's Top 50 Food Activists by the Academy of Culinary Nutrition.

Lari Laurikkala

Lari's passion for cooking became apparent during his childhood, when days spent foraging near his Finnish home always ended with him pulling his mother into the kitchen, eager to start cooking. As a teenager, Lari detoured from his culinary pursuits when he landed a role on Finland's most popular television show, *Salatut Elämät* (*Secret Lives*). The show opened him up to a world of adventure. Traveling around the world during his twenties, Lari found himself on a perpetual quest to try local foods and new ingredients. Eventually, he returned to cooking and opened a catering business focused on incorporating superfoods, Chinese herbal medicine, and Ayurvedic practices. Since its inception in 2012, Lari has acted as chef and product manager of Four Sigmatic.

CONVERSION CHART

All conversions have been rounded up or down to the nearest whole number.

Liquid Measures

US	MILLILITERS
1 teaspoon	5
2 teaspoons	10
1 tablespoon	14
2 tablespoons	28
¼ cup	56
½ cup	120
¾ cup	170
1 cup	240
1¼ cups	280
1½ cups	340
2 cups	450
2¼ cups	500, ½ liter
2½ cups	560
3 cups	675
3½ cups	750
3¾ cups	840
4 cups or 1 quart	900
4½ cups	1000, 1 liter
5 cups	1120

Weight Measures

OUNCES	POUNDS	GRAMS	KILOS
1		28	
2		56	
3½		100	
4	¼	112	
5		140	
6		168	
8	½	225	
9		250	¼
12	¾	340	
16	1	450	
18		500	½
20	1¼	560	
24	1½	675	
27		750	¾
28	1¾	780	
32	2	900	
36	2¼	1000	
40	2½	1100	1
48	3	1350	
54		1500	1½

Oven Temperature Equivalents

FARENHEIT	CELCIUS	GAS MARK	DESCRIPTION
225	110	¼	Cool
250	130	½	
275	140	1	Very Slow
300	150	2	
325	170	3	Slow
350	180	4	Moderate
375	190	5	
400	200	6	Moderately Hot
425	220	7	Fairly Hot
450	230	8	Hot
475	240	9	Very Hot
500	250	10	Extremely Hot